Golden-Tips for Humanity

Any person, group of persons or nation that in others' inspire harmony, will always move up ahead in this race for life; and will forever remain up there ahead, so long as their mindset remains unaltered; inversely, any person, group of persons or nation that in others stir up strife and friction will always move downwards and remain down in the same order of things. This is one of Nature's Golden Rules; that order will never be reversed so long as all the elements of creation remain the same; unaltered!

Evidently everything in the entire universe seems to be in peace and harmony with themselves except human relationship; why? Because, humans have not learnt to give freely without expecting to receive; they don't seem to have yet grasped the golden fact that, the more you give away freely, especially in service to others, the more you receive and of course, the richer you must become; in material and spiritual realm! Another Golden-Rule of Nature which in majority we seem to neglect in our day-to-day affairs with life in general; and of course, the results are obvious-colossal collapse and rapid degeneration of our vital force…

WHAT IS A REAL AND AN IDEAL LIFE FOR US?

As I sit writing this, I have clocked over five decades in this awesome world. And as I reminisce or look back without bias, I can effortlessly see the difference between forty to fifty years ago counting down to this day. The big difference which had been taking place from then till today is simply enormous and tear-jerking.

In my view, from what I've seen and known from then down to this day, I will prefer to live in this present time with the mindset of the past decades. Why do I say that or make such a choice irrespective of all the high technological advancement and ultra- modern civilization or growth in all facets of this present time? To answer that, I will like us to briefly and with mind eye assimilate the following basic issues, affairs that make each individual true human which are being forcefully eroded consciously or otherwise. That will prepare you for what follows

Comparing fifty years down to this day:

1. As a child from the early-sixties, I remember walking naked around our house and our neighborhood even at five or above without feeling shy or any form of quilt. Today, such natural feeling of innocence had been replaced with the ugly feeling of quilt and shyness under the same circumstance; why and what went wrong?
2. I remember also how both sexes of our communities used to swim naked amongst them: mothers and sons, fathers and daughters, all swimming and playing in the same river without shyness, quilt or any form of negative sentiments. Today, boys and girls of any age are not allowed to associate in any way possible for intimate interactions; what had gone wrong and when did that rupture took place?
3. I also remember as recent as the eighties, how we used to feel deep affection and sympathy for any of our family members to even neighbors when they are in pain from sickness or anything whatsoever abnormal on their ways. Today, we instead feel joy and apathetic if our family member or neighbor suffers and in pain; which, in most cases, in these days, we even do things with

the intention to bring direct pain and hardship to our own relatives.

4. As a child, I vividly remember how we used to constantly think of what to give, do for or help our direct family and community at adulthood. And, as soon as we reach adult and able, our first income or material gains goes to our beloved parents or brothers and sisters before we shall ever have the sense to think of doing anything for our own personal benefits. Today, hardly do I see or notice such virtue in anyway anywhere whatsoever. What happened? In place of such good deeds, most that I see are children who abuse and insult their parents up to even when they become adults; some accuse their parents of not doing one thing or the other for them; and no matter how much the parents had labored to cater for them, still they will take the offensive stance. If at adult in these days, a person is unsuccessful, there are always the parents' and the country to blame for his or her plight! Wow! What a great generation of humans that we very busy reproducing and educating? How shall we as people retrieve and revive our eroding and fading intrinsic values?

And what should an ideal system of government be for us?

After all said and done; at the end of the day; the daunting question still is: **'what is the essence of leadership for you? Is it to lead your people towards the protocol of: love, peace and harmony; as, to enable them savor the hidden benefits which are replete in the pathway to love, peace, and unity in harmony?**

Or *does true leadership mean to lead your obedient people: to war to kill and be killed; to hate and vandalize, cheat and deceive; leaving them with the sure repercussions such trait of character carry and distribute along with them?*

Whatever your personal answer may be to the above questions, I advise you to think it out well over before you decide and act.

But, for me, my candid view is that, every living being or thing has got just, two basic choices in their everyday life; and these two choices fundamentally determine their own essence of life; their character trait, their general concepts and choices of values. In our everyday lives, we are confronted with some looming obligations to do either this or that; to deny this or to accept that; to delete or to save; and to go or to stay…

If that is the immutable reality of our everyday lives, we are obliged to live with such constant moments of decision making and choice taking through to the very last of our respective days here on Earth! Take your decisions with prudence and act with caution.

In addition, this tricky question popped up from nowhere on my mental screen asking: **'after all said and done, in time to reckon and to give an account for the deeds and activities which we carried out when we have the liberty to decode and choose; what then for you, is the essence of life?**

Is it to spend most of your life in schools; at work and in desperate pursuit of material wealth and fame; with their inevitable negative repercussions? Or does life also mean for you: love, peace and harmony with yourself, family, neighbors, and other people; together with the things of creation in general; and the guaranteed benefits they carry along with them?

You presume and accepted that, 'your destiny is in your hands', why then must you obediently continue to do things which you are often asked to do; more than those things which you really would want to do, which are yearning and yelling for attention from your deeper mind? Before you answer, take a walk on one side; look inside out of you while you think it well over.

On the other hand, why then, have human race not been able to discover the protocol of: love, peace and harmony as we are cleverly advancing with Science and Technology; during this long history of our existence on 'Mother-Earth'?

In summary, to be able to govern or lead people smoothly, you must be able to learn to govern or lead first yourself; your family and friends toward finding: love, unity, peace and harmony. In the absence of learning to govern and lead yourself harmoniously, you can never be able to govern or lead others well enough to achieve: love, peace and harmony of which you were unable to achieve on your own. **These are the ultimate goals of all people; to find, during their lifetime: love, good health, wealth, peace and harmony!**

In a nutshell, it is obvious that, human beings, in the long history of their continued existence on this Earth have always had the freedom to decide and choose. But, sadly, I lack the knowledge of any era in these long histories of human race marked by this kind of: peace, love and harmony which I am making reference to in this book. **I refer to the kind of: love, peace and harmony which you can achieve only through the dint of hard inner-work; the looming task of 'deciding' and 'choosing' which begins and ends our everyday lives.** I, also, refer to the kind of: love, peace and harmony you alone can find, use and feel, for yourself alone through all your given organs: your sight, tongue, ears, nose and your central nervous system.

To be frank with you, from my years of experiences and understanding of the simple, but, complicated protocol of: love, peace, unity and harmony; and together with that of the Creation, I can stake anything that our global government or leadership system was designed and built on the wrong premise; therefore, our leadership is busy working pathetically on the wrong pathway to life and now, find themselves entangled in the mesh of complications, frustrations and dissatisfaction. Colossal collapse for disobeying Nature's Golden-Rules...

The global human attitude and conduct; the crisis, the wars and terrorism are some of the obvious manifestations of how far away we are distancing ourselves, our born and unborn children from the path leading to the only real things of this life: love, peace, unity and harmony which we are all wrongly searching for everyday in diverse and frenetic, if not ridiculous ways.

Fine! We need money because we designed money; all fine! **But, the hard knock questions are: for what do we really need this money, fame and all these material aggrandizement?** Are they to find and accumulate: love, peace, unity, good health and harmony or are they to seek and buy: Houses, food, clothes and fame? *Obviously, as I sit writing, we have for years sought and found: houses, food, clothes and caprices; but, have we equally found: love, peace, sound health and harmony in all these long years of human history?* Think this well over before you give your opinions.

The reality and an ideal life is really so simple that in most of our everyday lives, those real things that really matter so much to us, seem not to matter anymore; they often seem not to be there anymore. Whenever you take notice of your needs, desires and wellbeing seeming to be further away from you, don't panic; all your birthright and natural given potentials are still intact; they must remain intact because the rules which are binding all created things including you, are nearly infallible and incorruptible. You are only momentarily being confused for not knowing what are the right stances, and the right decision and action to take on the spur of the moment in order to keep you going; nothing is wrong or far away from your easy reach!

The crux of the whole matter is that, when you stop to nourish, appreciate and care for whatever you have, either from birth, given or acquired; automatically, you will gradually stop to take notice, savor or beneficially use those things around you that were duly created for your wellbeing; in and within the precinct of your present habitats.

Precisely, human race or our global communities are just exactly in the same rut; they are just being themselves.

To correct your unwanted situation, you must strive to float in harmony with the 'well thought over' decisions and choices oozing from the interior of your subconscious mind. Doing anything whatsoever contrary to the dictate of your mind, irrespective of the physical and momentary benefit does not render much benefit to you.

The decision you make and the action you take at any given moment of your life is synonymous with the life you live, and of that which you will keep living and giving; so, decide and act positive at all moments; that is your maximum security against unforeseen complications along the future as you progress in life.

Our main pledge here should be, to lead us towards the protocol of: unity, love, peace and harmony for the wellbeing and welfare of the entire global citizens as it is or should be in the legendary heaven!

INTRODUCTION

Obviously humanity is in full swing disarray and fortunately the way out, the way forward is deep-down-within us. Irrespective of wherever you are, your creed, gender or cultural background; I only want you to bear in mind that this world belongs to us all; is also governed by the rules and regulations of the Creator or what I call 'Creational-Rules'. That in context, we henceforth should stop taking to heart most of the "man-made-rules that direct and govern our individual lives. Every human is born with the inalienable right to decide and choose the best way forward in this world of infinity and spirituality. Every given life in this world is absolutely individualistic. But, fortunately also, the golden rules for unity and harmony in our individualistic designs are conspicuously coded in our mind's chip or "Mother-board" and the ignorance or sound knowledge of those facts, should not be an excuse to taunt and manipulate our humanistic birth rules. Above all that, the quintessential of "Creational Rules" is that, do what we may, we should for peace, unity and harmony sakes never ever infringe on anyone's right of choice and decision; once we do that, the natural system design of our individuality shall be jeopardized. In our leadership roles as the guardians of this planet Earth, are we complying with the above laws of our Maker/Creator?

To assert the veracity of that claim, let's consider why in all these countless years of human history – the sun continued to rise and set at regular periods; the rain continues to fall and cease; the moon continued to come and go; the stars, the cloud in continuous movement; the wind invisible and invincible but ever noticeable; the Ocean and the Earth remain ever in their mapped places; so, also, for all species of plants and animals including me and you, now and here today.

Our complicated and sophisticated reproduction and multiplication processes had ever remained unchanged and infallible; how could you explain all that marvel with the simple word of mouth or gesture of the body?

All of the above shows that there is clear orderliness in the creation and smooth running of every seen and conceivable thing in this world and those beyond. Like science and technology, the same sequence of rules, guidelines and regulations help to sustain their invented item to continue to work and function appropriately; and any of the components out of regulation will surely disrupt the smooth functioning of the said item. The entire universe functions in the same way; governed by rules and guidelines.

Based on this premise, I imagined that sound and superb human beings capable of versatility can be conscientiously raised by simply applying and following the same rules and regulations of the universal Creator starting from the day of our birth to the day we die.

All of the above serve only to show that there is celestial orderliness in all created matter and circumstances. Just in the same way that science and technology require rules and regulations to sustain the continuity of their inventions and discoveries; similarly, the Creator has rules and regulations for the infinite continuity of all created objects. With all that in mind, I coined together this unique "Blueprint for the "Leadership of Unity & Equity for Humanity" as the most feasible way forward. To achieve this feat is easy if only we can aim to consciously imitate the positive rules and regulations of the Creator in relation to: action/reaction, love/hate, give/take, work/pleasure… in a nutshell; to reduce most of the present and past global challenges daunting us and design a government based on "Leadership of Unity and Equality for Humanity", to achieve peace and harmony, we must have to live according to the guidelines given by the Creator deep-down-within us without adding and or subtracting.

On behalf of the mighty Creator of this world which I'm so deeply proud to be part of; on behalf of deepest love, sympathy and respect for entire creation (microcosm); on behalf of peace, harmony and unity, I present this proposal for a global political reshuffle in the best future ways our nations should be headed and managed as to sustain and uphold our good dreams to foster in harmony with the indomitable forces of Nature. All that we really need to live our given lives marvelously is simply by doing things in unity with our good conscience; and with love, peace and harmony…and in alignment with the forces of nature.

It therefore amazes me that to this day, at this very moment, we have made a lot of achievements and realized commendable feats in almost all aspects of our lives yet, we have not known for just one month in a row deep: peace, love, unity and harmony. Time for that is long overdue; let's give now, today a holistic try to realize ideal global peace, unity in harmony of which will bring equality for humans to contribute their fair quota of good will to each other without bias.

This book is based on one child's experiment with himself in search for the best way to live in peace and harmony with oneself, the environment and entire humanity; to cater for, protect and appreciate nature itself. That experiment continued to this child's adulthood and to this day; as this book is being written, he is still head to toe deeply immersed in his personalized methodologies for realizing endless flow of: love, peace, unity and harmony within the core of his innermost self which, surely, must function as well for our global communities'.

These endless personalized experiments have given this unknown child endless possibilities to live through nearly every human factor in first person experiences; such personalized experiences accumulated in the course of time, today, have come to form the building block and foundation stone for this book – "Humanity in Disarrays-The Ways Forward" and with the subtitle-"Leadership of Unity and Equity for Humanity". For the author, this book should be considered as the blueprint for "A REALISTIC GUIDELINES FOR GLOBAL CONSTITUTION"!

Inspired by deep respect for the Creator; the beauty and the infinity of beauty in most things of creation, unconditional love for humanity, every environment and the immensity of the mind-capacity…

His childhood dream was to see and live in a really united world where words are taken as bonds for what they really stood for from all human perspectives of word-use; a world without boundaries; a world where every human sees one another as brothers and sisters.

In honor to such inspiration, I have spent nearly my entire life searching for a more effective, viable and lasting solution to most human problems as they affect every one of us who are subjected directly or indirectly to human rules, from the past to the present.

I was very bitter growing up and seeing the high degree of chaos and disharmony in human system of things. I could not understand why human systems give too much energy pushing and pursuing things that do not encourage peace and harmony. In adulthood, I discovered to my dismay the fact that, mankind is seriously acting and being governed by ignorance of the true way to live the best of nature. I had to forgive them and kept seeking for a more viable and durable solution to the globalized human problems…

Ladies and gentlemen, children and youth, I solemnly invite you to embrace this book as your blueprint for a 'New Guideline for World Constitutional reshuffling' for the true leadership of unity and equality for entire humanity; for peace and harmony to reign supreme!

You have no problem that cannot be resolved by the immense power of your innermost mind if you are privileged to reach it and harmonize with it. All we need is a good and honest guidance from our leaders or from those privileged to know the appropriate and accurate attitude to life, which comes through grind and hard-earned experiences.

Global crisis!

A nation, like a person, to be truly successful and prosperous, must be able to at least, set-out short-term and long-term goals; upon which, the nation's or person's entire life should oscillate or pivot; the short-term goals will serve as a compass which will guide and guard the person or nation through across the vast oceans, space and time in order to achieve and embrace the set-out long-term goal! Without that, the nation or person becomes a puppet for the Spirits; a pendulum dangling from left to right, front to back and vice versa. That is the major problem with most nations as with most people of this awesome world; living without set-out goals; living aimlessly and hopelessly and Crisis of all kinds becomes our reward

What therefore is or had been our collective global goal pursuit? None!

How global crisis?

Certainly there is global economic, social, political, religious crisis etc. Fine! I agree with you; with all the cliché, but, the inevitable question is-

What solution did you suggest, suggested or suggesting that will or may help to make things of our world function better than how it is now and or have been before?

The majority of us are very good talkers; and therefore, can criticize with ease; but without giving any simple or viable solution to any of the abundant and lingering human problems; not even capable to solve their own immediate family and personal problems.

I heard you say 'there is a solution to every problem' **why then are our crisis and other global problems continued to ascend geometrically instead of diminishing progressively?**

From the obviously precarious nature of things of creation, especially, in direct relationship with human entities, don't you think it's become more urgent than ever before to start doing something positive and proactive with an aim to design a new global order of things; global order or rules designed to change the human mindset from the present habit of embracing negative attitudes more quicker in place of positive mental attribute. I believe it's inevitably time to change our wrong global beliefs in many things of creation and incline consciously toward doing only what is right and just!

The truth is there is no problem with this world or about creation itself. The problem is all inside our mind and our mind's configurations; therefore to effectively combat the looming global challenges, we must attune our mindset to harmonize with the due changes we wish to make outwardly.

This book is all about new and practical ways to live in, harmonize with, and manage the affairs of the entire universe to the very best ever.

How shall that be achieved?

That could be done simply by- *applying with appreciation and enthusiasm the concept of the 'Golden-rules of Mother-Nature.* This is the only viable gateway for a positive new beginning! The only way that will make it possible for us to consciously walk the arduous road back to nature for the abundant wealth and benefits it offers.

Enough of shortcuts in life! We want to begin to witness brotherhood and sisterhood in our neighborhoods; where peace, unity and harmony will reign for a long time! That long awaited change is finally here! This book with its contents must bring that long awaited global mind-sweep for the best changes ever. Yes we can, so let's just do it!

WAY FORWARD
World Citizenship Identification Card –WCIC-
To begin this race for global unification, all humans at their birth should be given as usual, a name for identification purposes in time of need. With the help of Google map and others, we will devise a centralized global leadership system that will permit those in charge of global affairs to see live occurrences of what is happening in the streets of every corner of the entire globe; identify each family by face and name. People will carry electronic gadget with chip that can connect them direct to the central global representative of their area or region for any form of issue bothering them, whenever they are in need of quick and prompt solution or aid; even in time to take decisive action, if they will not be sure what to do and how to do it, all they need do is: just connect to their given transmission gadget that will link them to the central body of their area and get immediate and sincere advice from the horses' mouth, on one-to-one, and directly without any "bullshit" or bureaucratic impediment.

No more wars; no more fighting; now is the time for global peace and harmony; yes we can achieve if we believe!

Sample Draft of the- WORLD CITIZENSHIP IDENTIFICATION CARD –WCIC-

-Place of origin… World Citizen

-Name… Amaechi

-Surname… Obi

-Place of birth… Ugbelle (city name) /Africa

-Date of birth… 1965

-Expiring date…none (permanent)

I purposely refused to include the country name of a person's birth, because, I strongly believe that, with this new system of global unification, there will be no more need for such words as: "My country" in place of that, we will get used to saying "my place of birth" or "city name". We are now of one globe; one world… let's copy from the rest of the animal creatures; we are one of them. What makes you think you are better or wiser than: dogs, goats, birds etc.? We are just another kind of specie; but not better or worse, just another kind of specie; get these issues very clear within your mindset!

You must be able to see the world and yourself in this way to understand the futility of all the ado, stress and material aggrandizement which we ignorantly chose to embark upon in this pretty world.

"United we will stand stronger and happier; divided as we are, we will fall and continue to shatter"

NO MORE WARS; NO MORE FIGHTING!

NOW IS THE ERA FOR GLOBAL PEACE AND HARMONY

NOW IS TIME TO CHANGE FOR THE BEST EVER LIVED OR SEEN

YES WE CAN; WE HAVE ALL THE REQUISITES FOR THE BEST CHANGES EVER KNOWN OR WITNESSED IN OUR LONG HISTORY.

PIECE OF ADVICE TO GLOBAL COMMUNITY

Whenever you learn to live your respective lives in conformity or in harmony with the 'Golden Rules' or 'Creational Laws' of Mother-Nature; or when you are more inclined to positive mental attitude, you will truly discover for yourself that the most you give or dish-out, the more you are bound to receive in equal or more proportion. No single living or even a non living entity that hasn't got anything to offer or receive in return. Why is this so? Because, every single created matter or element is usually ingrained with all the ingredients they will need to survive and make a successful living for themselves, and also, more than enough to give away; Life is sharing, giving and receiving.

In that premise, you will discover that no one or thing do actually give away anything for nothing; whenever we give to others, for example, what you are doing in that moment you think you gave something away, is actually getting something back for future use; it is like saving for the future ahead. We really do not do anything for people, but, rather, for ourselves; you can't educate someone else other than yourself; you can't work for people but for yourself. Every action attracts automatic reaction which is far beyond our control...

Each time you do a job for a company or for a boss, you are actually working or doing the job for yourself. You are obviously learning and acquiring knowledge which is what real life without money is all about! "Doing something and learning something"

Similarly, due to our erroneous interpretations of many issues of life, most entrepreneurs remain with the illusion that people are working for them; why? Because of the stupid money issues in between; no sir/s, you are the one actually working for those people under you! You are helping or showing them to earn a living through following your instructions and directives. Also, because you are assumed to be the first who initiated and been doing much for the growth of the business in question; you have done and are still doing the same job before others can follow up in order to later take over from you as the boss and give back to you in gratitude; you are expending effort to share that knowledge which you have worked hard to acquire!.. This same principle applies in all things of life including: political, religious and academic leaderships etc.

What then is leadership if not serving others; showing them what you have done and how to achieve the same successful result you are supposed to have achieved before then?

What is leadership other than service with unconditional love to others and things of creation in general?

What is work other than thought which is put into action for an ingathering for oneself, others and things in general?

However, if you are able to grasp that simple universal principle, you will as well be able to grasp what is wrong with our global community in direct relationship with humanity as whole; and not with yourself alone; your issues are not unique but, universally designed!

However, to add to that, it is in no way economical or better, to fret to search for a remedy after causing enormous damages to fellow humans and to things of creation; it is best to fret most to avoid embarking on such damaging projects or actions from the start…

Not for nothing our ancestors noted that: "prevention was better than the cure" for example- the recurring issues of cigarettes, alcohol, addictive drugs, nuclear weapons, silicone implants; and manufacture of plastic bags, racial discrimination and immigration issues etcetera. Those are products with side effects and socially controversial.

The questions are: does it mean we humans are not clever enough to know beforehand the after effects or consequences of the actions we embark upon; or that we cannot be bothered to assume responsibilities for actions we take or the damages that we do to other humans and to the things of creation in general?

Or do you think and feel that, money and material benefits are more important than the mass damages you do to global citizens, ecosystem and entire works of art of the Creator?

Global inventors and discoverers, please fret more when considering the long term benefits of all your inventions for your fellow global citizens; consider meticulously, the long term advantages and disadvantages of your every invention before offering them for public use. Authorizing bodies also endeavor to consider the advantages and disadvantages to the global community before you fret to authorize any of your products for use. This way we can collectively fret to prevent than fret to cure!

DEDICATION

To my beloved world; to the Creator of all these wonders everywhere you maybe or have the privilege to visualize! To unity, Love; Peace and Global Harmony! To Wisdom; as the foundation Stone for the entire Human Reality! To my beloved wife and family!

WHAT IS GLOBALIZATION?

-In Wikipedia globalization is presented as follows-:

"Globalization refers to the increasing unification of the world's economic order through reduction of such barriers to international trade as tariffs, export fees, and import quotas. The goal is to increase material wealth, goods, and services through an international division of labor by efficiencies catalyzed by international relations, specialization and competition. It describes the process by which regional economies, societies, and cultures have become integrated through communication, transportation, and trade. The term is most closely associated with the term economic globalization:

the integration of national economies into the international economy through trade, foreign direct investment, capital flows, migration, the spread of technology, and military presence. [1] However, globalization is usually recognized as being driven by a combination of economic, technological, socio-cultural, political, and biological factors. [2] The term can also refer to the transnational circulation of ideas, languages, or popular culture through acculturation. An aspect of the world which has gone through the process can be said to be **globalized"**.

-Globalization is, in addition to the above definition, a positive and proactive project truly extending its tentacles to the remotest, most forgotten places of the world. Globalization is a positive shift in the human mindset aiming at replacing the old order of things, which allowed and permitted, few privileged persons or nations to manage the affairs of other people in matters relating to: economy, politics, and technology, socio-cultural and biological. With humanity desiring to unite their efforts and activities as a nation in one, as brothers and sisters pursuing a common objective for the sincere benefit of all people of the globe, the result is already very positive and continue to sensitize a good number of nations into setting up proactive plans and actions aimed at realizing this goal on a grand scale! Our entire world shall then be globalized when all nations join hands and speak with a unanimous voice in favor of these global pursuits and challenges founded in peace and harmony.

WHAT IS THE BEST STRATEGY TO ACCELERATE MASS AWARENESS TO THESE IMPENDING GLOBAL CHALLENGES?

CNN with such programs as: 'Global Challenges,' 'Go Beyond Borders'. BBC with 'Hard Talk' and many other Media contributions all around the world, 'Global Exchange', other NGO and private individuals are strongly in the forefront doing and using everything within their means to spread information, initiate positive actions, identify and localize the problems and then, call for actions. These corporations and individuals are already taking the lead in surmounting most of the identified dangers threatening lives, peace and harmony; my special thanks and unreserved respect to all those people who are dedicating their energy for the common good of this rich world and inhabitants.

Globalization, to make a durable impression that will positively impart and impact on the citizens of this rich world, we must hurry to devise an effective method which will help to slowly attune the mindset of all persons to a reasonable level of awareness of themselves and their environment to an intimate relationship.

Leadership by example is another effective way to inculcate a globalized ideology into the mindset of world citizens through living and doing, with conviction and enthusiasm; doing things that we judge and accept as correct.

Globalization must be concentrated on gaining the unbiased attention of everybody inside this globe, teaching them without reservations the simplest ways to maintain positive mental attitudes at all times towards every single thing of creation.

More appropriately, include and inculcate the globalization ideology into the main stream of our academic curriculum. This should be a positive indoctrination with a huge advantage- involving entire humanity to consciously work towards a collective goal for substantive future rewards aimed at benefiting our global environment, people and all nations!

Children must be fully involved from the start of these projects. They are the key; the main target for the true impact of globalization to be driven safely home. Our children all over the world should be made to embrace the utmost importance of those issues challenging their future security. The aim will be to open the minds of our children to the challenges looming ahead of them, and the best ways to tackle those challenges for the benefit of all global communities and citizens.

The children should be educated to assimilate these correct senses of ideal values, put them into practice as they grow into adulthood; the end result shall be: nations full of men and women prepared and motivated to consciously do things right. Do things; take initiatives and actions that will benefit most people than just a few as in the present dispensation of 'things of the world'

Finally, for globalization to sink well and settle down in peoples' minds, spark the engine of true global consciousness forceful enough to motivate world citizens to voluntarily cater for their environments as they do cater for their homes and material properties; when we could do those, then the job will already be halfway done.

One-on-one with this project, we must direct our people to be aware that: we are all brothers and sisters, that this rich world collectively belongs to all of us; this world is our home, our heaven, paradise and hell… that wherever they find their selves is their home at that moment and should be duly catered for! These are some of the ways forward in the right path.

That to find peace, enjoy their given lives, they must practice catering and nurturing for their respective environments. That every hidden damage they do to plants, forests, animals, humans, lands, seas and the atmosphere transforms into a potential danger with the passage of time; which will affect and inflict innocent people in negative ways. Common examples of such repercussions of wrong doings include: global economic crisis, persistent drought and the misery it spreads along, environmental contamination and its adverse effects, deforestation and its toll on live and wide-stocks, global warming and rampant earthquakes. On the other hand: racism, discrimination, mass ignorance, mass corruption etc. There is no end to the list of challenges facing us ahead, but, we can easily surmount them all if we join minds and hands together as one people under the same roof! Then, and only then will the word 'globalization', its meaning and benefit come to live with us as an inseparable part and parcel of our lifestyle – love, peace, unity in harmony, wealth and joy will be there for all to take home and enjoy without fear and uncertainty!

LEADERSHIP OF UNITY & EQUITY FOR HUMANITY
-Blueprint for a Viable Globalization-

As a living person, I can confess that somehow, I cope well enough with life within my confines; and to the best of my abilities, I am living out my dearest life in: Peace, unconditional Love and Harmony amidst these ceaseless global conflicts and unfavorable challenges. *Sure, Peace, Love and Harmony are sensations of vital energy forces deep-down-within each one of us.*

But to awaken those vital energy forces to take predominance of our dearest everyday life, make them work for us, in our favor through their constant supply of vital energy forces to us; which, if maintained and allowed free flow will usually engulf us with the sensation of wellbeing; which shall then be expressed in optimism, enthusiasm and gratitude for life; for that to happen in us, we must work hard for it! To live with peace, love and harmony, you must sacrifice hard for it. You must have to discover and know yourself well enough through conscious adventure, fall and rise.

In a nutshell, to live your dear lives in peace, with love and in harmony with yourselves and your environments, you must have a burning desire for general knowledge; you must be humble with the burning desire to learn and enough time for you alone to meditate on a daily basis all through your life! (Every second counts).

However, you may accomplish with all of the above prerequisites, but, without the constant exuberance in positive mental attitude streamlined within all your daily affairs, the core Peace, Love and Harmony may not duly manifest in some cases. That, also, is the crux of the matter!

I have in addition equally questioned: the Creator, the Devil, the Leaders, the Parents, the teeming people and friends along my life's journey; but, unfortunately, without receiving cogent answers to these looming and pervading global challenges. I cannot stop worrying for my beloved world; so much that, I am worn-out. Neither could I stop being angry for the ways humans around the globe seem to be gratefully misleading one another. Nevertheless, out of my obvious frustrations and worries, I received this 'Divine Inspiration' structured in the only most viable way to better the lives of every global citizen in this current race for desperate search for short-term remedies to the near everlasting issues of life.

For me, I had for long chosen to dedicate my entire life to learn, and searching incognito mostly from within me the charm, beauty and mystery of the phenomena humans and their environment in my reach; and to my dismay and chagrin, I discovered that about ninety percent of what we term Global Problems' are duly caused by humans themselves!

Other questions occurred out of this shocking discovery:

What are the reasons why humans cause problems; create confusions and frustrating circumstances for themselves? Is it out of ignorance or out of malice? This topic should be open for global debate, but, for me, I will suffice to assume that most people decide and act out of **-Ignorance-** in dealing with themselves and their everyday affairs. Ignorance simply means: having little or no knowledge of things, situations or circumstances. Why do I choose to accept that most global citizens decide and act governed by ignorance; why that choice?

Because, for me, maliciousness is a remote sign of ignorance; to act with malice or any other way other than, ways that are universally accepted, and those which must foster peace and harmonious co-existence amongst humans and their environment, tantamount to the unawareness of the lurking consequences on equal ratio to the level of thought and action taken at that spur of the moment. These factors represent some of the subtle laws of nature which, usually beacon the ways positively forward for us all. Therefore, not doing things right means that one is ignorant of the best practices or that one is intentionally acting with the wish or desire to do wrong or harm to others or to things.

- I wonder what kind of human spirit could act with such malice; unless, the legendary story of the 'Devil or Satan' deriving pleasure out of peoples' distresses is true. Nevertheless, otherwise, I had comfortably chosen to say that: *majority of humans are truly ignorant of what life and living is all about.*

Based on that premise, I had come up with the only durable and viable solution to all global human problems if we can all agree to agree to work things out proactively.

All the human life's mechanism is coordinated deep down within their respective minds. So, by balancing the equations of our respective minds, we can then balance the rhythms or equations of our respective lives; so doing, we can be able to achieve: Peace, love, unity in harmony on a global perspective. There is no known magic or easier way out in

the right...

The following are my lines of thought and action which, without doubt, if duly respected and applied by all global nations and citizens, shall make it possible for us to achieve that global objective which is – a leadership system bound in unity and equity for all humanity- a better world for all and sundry is our next global pursuit after years of senseless wars, scramble for wealth, domination and fake supremacy over other citizens and nations... for unity and peace sake, we must reshuffle and reset our individual minds to align with the Golden-Rules of life; and that is as simple as we need do to reach our "Promised-Land"

There are multi-facets to achieve unity and peace under a proactive leadership structure which must start step-by- step as stipulated with the foundation of an education system for some chosen children from all nooks and corners of any sovereign nation in the world...

INSTITUTE FOR GLOBAL PEACE AND HARMONY- IGPH

Down the line of human history from time immemorial, there never had been an era marked with peace, love, unity and harmony; in its place had always been: brutal wars, massacres, supremacy, tribalism, and nationalism; and most recent is discrimination, all forms of phobia, terrorism and fanatics. Why not the other way round? Are these supposed to be the true nature of humankind? Or was something wrong along the line of creation? These whole issues of wars, killing of one another, betrayals, cheating, and discrimination of fellow man and woman never seize to deeply challenge my scope of imagination.

I do not want to go into details of all the personal troubles I was subjected to from childhood seeing these negative human conducts against each other; especially, intuiting and with the deepest feeling that, we could do much better than all that. As a result of that deepest feeling to see and live in a world where: love, peace, unity and harmony reign supreme, I became irresistibly inspired to coin together and portray this piece of proposal as the only viable avenue for global peace, unity and harmony.

Certainly, you will wonder what gave me the authority and braveness to delve into this 'sacred topic'. You will find your answer in my first and endless book -**Universal Child**- I truly had paid my dues to the Creator, to Satan and to the human-made-system all to my own peril. And based on all the challenges, my blind adventures and fights to remain afloat in this daunting ocean of life today as I sit writing, I strongly belief that I have known enough of myself and that of entire human mind-set which is making it possible for me to write this piece of proposal which I am duly presenting to you accordingly in the following easy steps:

-IGPH- Institute for Global Peace and Harmony

For any viable and proactive change to be made or effected in this world today as it is, a global change of mental attitude towards all created matters must have to be the first step ever. Humankind must be made to use or shown to apply what we term as: "POSITIVE MENTAL ATTITUDE" (PMA) in all their daily affairs; in relation with one another and when conducting any kind of business with each other. And to learn and to acquire anything tangible and valuable out of nature, that we must have or know, "POSITIVE MENTAL ATTITUDE" still remains the "DIVINE-KEY" Without the full understanding and application of the potentials of PMA in all our respective actions and reactions, the content in this book will be rendered worthless because the entire book content is founded on that premise.

IGPH is an institution of learning whose students will act as 'the sacrificial Lambs' who will shoulder with the burden to learn, live and act in accord with the 'Golden Rules of Creation', of which PMA is the major subject and then shall later write or rewrite a practical and realistic 'New World Constitution' that will be based on their testimony of the authenticity of those everlasting and time proven Universal Laws which they have being appropriately coached and soundly taught during their fifteen years of study in –IGPH-

What is the major objective of IGPH?

The major aim of the IGPH will be to educate those children chosen from all the sovereign nations of the world; show them the meaning, the importance and best practices in all human circumstances streamlined within the creational rules of Mother-Nature. The chosen children from this exercise will therefore act as the beacon for all mankind to achieve and realize that state of mindset necessary for the kind of global change which will aim to benefit our global community in general irrespective of race, creed or gender.

How do we kick-start this level of global project?

Simple! All we need to do is select four brilliant children, between the ages of: four, five and six, from every sovereign country in this world; the children must be in the ratio of two boys to two girls out of each nation. The selection must be of uniform criterion and carried out only by unanimously appointed individuals; with an impeccable love for this world deep down their hearts. I will direct and see to the solid foundation and operation of the school.

In the similar way also, the schools' staffs and teachers shall be selected and groomed to the required level of understanding of the Golden rules of the Creator'.

The media, as always, owe full responsibility for making this good news reach out to every home and jungle around the four corners of the globe; from the world leaders down to the peasants, and to the domestic and jungle animals; whomsoever that can hear, see and understand should be made to know that- the entire world is voluntarily embarking on this very project of global change to the best ever; for peace, unity and harmony to reign supreme everywhere in replacement of the present system of wars, fighting and killing!

To truly initiate this mega-project, we will best start stage-by-stage:

STAGE - 1

-SELECTION OF CHILDREN AND STAFFS FOR IGPH-

IGPH will be made up of children between the tender ages of five to six years and will be fished out or selected from around the four corners of our globe by a special group of people or staffs who in turn will be chosen unanimously to carry out the selectivity exercises. The Said group of people or staffs will have to come together, sit and work out among themselves, a uniform plan for a smooth and impartial process at the time to select the ideal children for the –IGPH-

All sovereign countries must have to present a minimum of two children (a boy and a girl) and a maximum of four children (two boys and two girls) irrespective of creed, country or cultural background.

The type of people that will make up the group who will be responsible for selecting the pioneer students must be experts in the field of human psychology, Authors of successful self help books and some acclaimed clergymen/women of God and some "honest Media Gurus".

Those who shall scout and select the pioneer students shall be searching for such children who are less prone to negative influences; reference being made to every child's family-background and immediate habitat at the time of selection shall be paramount.

STAGE- 2

SELECTION OF STAFFS FOR IGPH

As I said earlier, the communication media should play the most important role in information dissemination through: the web, television stations, radio stations and newspapers, etcetera.

This institution will be staffed by people with faith and belief that, this vision and mission can easily be achieved. The school's staffs must have enviable and disciplined personal lifestyles; we will verify their profile and testimony from their closest neighbors. The chosen staffs for IGPH must be of positive attitude in most of their respective daily affairs and activities.

It will be preferable for this institution to be mostly staffed by authors of self-help books, psychologists, and people who are already showing concern and giving their efforts to similar services which are aiming to bettering this world's citizens and their respective environment.

To endorse or approve who stays as staff and who stays as student will finally be decided by the author of this book for some divine reasons...

STAGE – 3

LOCATION FOR IGPH

The stage three and final phase before the commencement of the project will be the location of the institution.

The global citizens shall unanimously have to decide on the most viable and effective location and modus operandi suitable for the school's aims and objectives. We will suffice here to have an idea of what –IGPH- students will be expected to realize in our collective world after their graduation that will be taking place between when they have attained the ages of- fifteen to twenty years.

STUDENTS' ASSIGNMENTS AFTER EDUCATION FROM IGPH

-Promulgation of Global Constitution and Leadership Strategy-

IGPH-students will be assumed ready for their assignments at the ripe ages of twenty. At such ages, they must have spent about fifteen years of intensive practical coaching aimed at applying those moral codes we consider the best intrinsic human values which work in harmony with creational rules for the achievement and realization of peace, unity and harmony for all global citizens and with other living and non-living species of creation; as well as conscientious care for our global atmospheric environment.

It will be expected that IGPH students must have mastered the importance of applying positive mental attitude in all affairs concerning humanity and their ecosystem; the true and ideal meaning of terms as: Leadership (service by example), definite purpose, success and failure, and above all, the advantage of applying a positive mental attitude and the disadvantage of also, applying a negative mental attitude in all human affairs; mastermind alliance and the enormous value of harnessing the efforts of more people in pursuit of a definite goal. When we have ascertained beyond reasonable doubt the soundness and positive impact on the quality of education imparted to those selected children, that will be the moment to set them free, let them loose to go for the divine mission of positive global change for which they have worked hard for, during their fifteen years of tenure in the IGPH!

STUDENTS BACK TO THEIR RESPECTIVE NATIONS TO RULE

Under a specific or special arrangement, each student will now be allowed to go back to their respective countries after completing the age of between: eighteen and twenty years under the impeccable and realistic training off -IGPH-

On the students' arrivals to their respective countries, all formalities will be carried out to receive them officially by each of their nations according to their customs and traditions.

In my opinion, I should suggest that said ex-students of IGPH should be received back home with open hands and seen as 'CHOSEN AND ANNOINTED PEOPLE'.

The next step will be to immediately hand over the leaderships of every global nation to them with the unanimous support of the people and by the people.

Out of the four selected children from each of the global nations, the first choice to head or lead any of their countries shall have to be, the female gender among them; and then, be assisted by their male colleagues. The rest of the graduates from the IGPH should be assigned to head the other branches of the government that are considered delicate or prone to corruption.

On an appointed date, all the prospective new or 'experimental' leaders will be globally sworn into office; and with that, the hallmark of a new era in the history of mankind!

COMMENCEMENT OF PROACTIVE LEADERSHIP

To commence duties officially, a couple of meetings and world conventions will have to be arranged in any chosen country and given location to discuss and bring into perspective all urgent matters which are in majority negatively affecting the world in general. And also, to review and design a standard system with which, each leader will have to use as a parameter to execute his or her leadership assignments.

There are many fundamental issues which must have to be addressed and tackled; with the main aim to trigger the wheels of peace, unity and harmony all around the world! From my personal analysis of creation in general, conscious and unconscious experiments carried out incognito I can pinpoint some of the major causes of global unrest from time immemorial to this present day.

In my view and to the best of my ability, for any leadership to bring unity and equality for all humanity, I have painstakingly compiled a list in order of importance, for most of the issues which need to be reviewed and corrected with urgency for this world to move further forward and to function smoothly on a positive perspective.

The issues listed below are paramount on my list of global challenges hindering peace and harmony in this world; from the past to this present day. We will have to face these challenges with the help of this 'new and honest constitution' for the betterment of humanity! There will include: reason, why, and how those new laws could foster global unity, peace and harmony when applied effectively and appropriately in our global political system.

To better this awesome world, among all the requisites, the first issue in my scale of preference is – **Language-**

LANGUAGE

-UNIFORM LANGUAGE FOR ALL NATIONS-

A dictionary defines language as "The particular form of sound or words used by a nation or group"

Taking the above definition into perspective, and applying the natural rules of things of creation, in all essence; it becomes imperative that a **common language** for all nations be carved-out, to compliment this new order of things. A uniform language for every global-citizen will help to form the nucleus, the engine and wheel of unity, equality and oneness among humanity.

The Creator Himself did a very good job in the classification of the living and nonliving matter into species. And each specie flocks together in respect for the natural law of 'like species flocking together', as it is for fishes, ants, birds' etcetera. So should it be also for humankind as common and unique specie amongst others. Therefore, it will be in the best interest of humankind to devise a common language for all humans in order to help bind them more closely together. This sense of togetherness cannot fail to maximize the global positive energy for peace and progress; success and harmony.

Don't you always feel very embarrassed when you are unable to communicate with fellow human in another corner of the globe? Do you enjoy that feeling of frustration when you cannot express yourself in front of someone when you are out of your corner of the globe? I doubt any sane person will like to be embarrassed in these kinds of situations.

The good news is that, such circumstances can easily be rectified just by **making all world citizens to speak the same language!**

To be realistic, as humans, the entire global citizens are supposed to use one particular form of sound or words to really make them feel like one in a family.

It is obvious that the use of a common language is the principal factor that identifies and unifies people as a race or a tribe.

If humans as unique or same specie could speak the same language, neighborhood and brotherhood will surely foster; plain understanding and acceptance of one another surely must foster; tribalism, discrimination and racial sentiments will gradually fade away and die a natural death.

The aim of this mission is to bring a durable change in the human mindset; teach all citizens of this great world, to think and act positive for a long time; this will make all of us better humans that will definitely transform our world into a better place for all to live and enjoy!

Enough of the old system of leadership and politics; this old system of things has continued from the beginning to hinder, hamper and jeopardize all global possibilities of: peace, love, unity and sense of brother/sisterhood. Time is over-due to fix all these situations negatively pervading the minds of global citizens and their environment.

In perspective to the complex global problems, **common language for all global citizens** among others should be the first universal or global assignment for the ex- students of the 'Institute for Global Peace and Harmony' IGPH.

HOW DO WE ELECT GLOBAL REPRESENTATIVES?

We must all sit round a very long table with food and drink to discuss how to carve-out or create a language every world citizen must have to speak, write and understand. From the look of things in the world as I write, we urgently need to find a way possible and easier for all human species to learn to make the **'same sound and speak the same word'**. When humanity or global citizens are able to speak a common language among them; read and write it in real time; then, that positive sense of oneness that nothing else could bring so far for now, shall then be made possible! Being able to speak the same language shall also promote that much sort after sensation of: love, peace, unity and equality in a way never before ever seen in the long history of this awesome world!

Secondly, in my list of factors negatively affecting global unity, peace and harmony is **'Money'- Money** stands strong as the second most urgent factor to be tackled and restructured in the best possible ways to put it in its rightful place in our lives.

Do not ever forget that, Money is only some pieces of synthesized paper with engraved mind-blowing, ingenious artistic designs of personalized color tricks; while on the other hand, the coins that compliment the paper money, is just some pieces of fused metals, carved out in varying denominations, designed and stamped and dispensed by our honorable men in 'BLACK'.

The only real value that all kinds of monies may have or have is only to the extent we respectively give our values to it; in order word, 'the real value of Money is that which we give to it'. Other than that, money will remain like any other item as paper and metal coins of no significance!

Do not give so much of your precious time in pursuit of money or other wealth or things that add so little to your state of mental and physical equilibrium or long time harmony. The rule of life is that, where most of your energy goes is where your heart will be in most of your everyday time. And, unfortunately, when you spend most of your precious time with fear and in desperate pursuit of money or external wealth, you will definitely suppress the yearning and yelling of your soul 'internal wealth' for attention.

If you ever desire to live long to satisfactorily reap the fruit of your labor with love, health, wealth with harmony; with peace and unity; then, you must have to reconsider your present decisions and choices. Think it out well over. But, nevertheless, with my hard-knock experiences, in my candid view, I will suggest that you give most of your precious time to the yearning and yelling of your 'internal wealth', your soul for your good and that of everyone around you. The ugliest aspect of this whole issue with money and material aggrandizement had sadly been that, 'the more wealth you accumulate, the more strain and stress you will also be complemented with. You cannot manipulate natural feelings or sensations because; their roots and sources are beyond our external link.

After all said and done, the crux of the entire issue of life and living-style, is that, every single organ or cell that work with us to keep us alive, definitely require care and attention which will only be possible to give if we make time to attend to their needs in reciprocal; making quality time to yourself alone is the pathway or gateway to the protocol of: love, wealth, happiness, peace and harmony structured in unity! Take your time and think it out well over; you will understand why you are unhappy with all your wealth and why the world is in crisis; when you think it out well over, you may come to the same or a better analysis and conclusion than I have put forward!

MONEY

USE OF COMMON-CURRENCY FOR ALL NATIONS

The question is can all global citizens design and use the same currency? My answer is capital- YES!

What shall be the economic and social effect of using a common currency in all global communities? Using common currency in all global communities definitely shall be the best thing that can ever happen to the human race now and after! They must have more unity, love, peace and harmony and equality. Life will suddenly for them become more meaningful; oh yeah! It must surely be.

From the look of things, money has gradually and systematically found its way into the mainstream of the entire human-race and hijacked their natural sense of sound reasoning; making them think and judge only of and in money; acting for money, working for money and ultimately living all their precious life for money! Today, in the more modern era of the long history of mankind, as I write money stands as a 'sine qua non to life on its own for modern people. These days, nearly every human-being thinks and believes that he or she must first have to make money in order to be able to live a 'real life'. Recently, this has become a global assumption. And without doubt, this very negative notion is instigating most people to perpetrate the majority of the anti-social and current heinous conducts pervading and overwhelming the present generation of the human race.

As language, money stands firm as the second most important weapon that can be applied to enhance -en-mass, the unity of all mankind as people in love and at peace with one another. On the contrary; the same money possesses the power to disintegrate and tear humanity apart as enemies under the same roof.

What are the advantages of all nations to use a common currency?

Use of **common currency for all nations** will:

- Help to unify mankind as one family inhabiting in different and diverse geographical locations.

- It will help to globalize most human aims and objectives, allowing people the possibilities to have similar good dreams and goals which will favor global interests.

- It will encourage world citizens to sincerely desire to work together with enthusiasm toward the same goal and also, making use of a standard parameter to conceive, believe and achieve those set goals.

- It will surely limit or mitigate most of the current and surging immigration and emigration challenges.

-Use of common currency in all the cities of the global communities will help to encourage the majority of the global youth who are prematurely leaving their places of origin together with their manpower which should have been used in improving their respective places of origin around the world; instead of abandoning their given places of origin to wither; while they go in hunt for bigger and easier money wherever they think will be best for them to grab it.

Embarking on such adventures will always bring to you: illusion and disillusion; these are feelings that will constantly dawn on you as you move ahead in your respective adventures, under man-made-rules. So, all your money pursuits will always turn out be 'just vain pursuits'.

Money, they say "is the root of all evil"- do you agree to that cliché? Money is not the evil itself; appropriate use of it either. It is, rather, the bedrock upon which lots of good and bad intentions and actions can well be made manifest.

The major problem in this context is 'not about having money or not having it', the major problem is that the perpetrators or inventors of the use of money, have had in their original intentions; they never made it for all to have it with ease and on equal backgrounds. It had always been a case of the 'winner taking it all' irrespective of what happens to the rest of the citizens; whether they live or die, that never bothered them. In fact, it was preferable if majority suffered and died for the few to have more money and

Too complicated for me to imagine and digest how sane people could invent things that create so excessive stress to obtain and own as it is with money.

I want to assure you that, you can always live comfortably well enough anywhere, with or without money; if you only know how to apply the 'Golden-Rules of Life' in all your daily affairs. Money is not created, but invented; therefore, can never be greater than anything created by the Creator as to deserve all that attention and sacrifices dedicated to its search and obtaining.

Now, having seen a few of the numerous advantages of using a **common currency for all nations;** let's briefly look at the various disadvantages of not using a **common currency for all nations:**

Money they say: 'is the root of all evil', why that age long belief? Simply because every bad or unacceptable activity taking place in the entire world from the past to the present day, had always been for the sake of Money or the desire to make money and possess more fame; as well as, more material things.

Money therefore, happens to be the major factor causing most of the simple and heinous crimes in all parts of the world today, such as: armed robbery with intimidation, hijacking, kidnapping, human and drug trafficking, prostitution and pornography, betrayals; and corruption etcetera. The majority of the global family problems today are all directly or indirectly connected to money. So also are the global wars and political unrest; all linking to money.

Frankly, it is far beyond my human imagination to think of the reason why nothing had been done in all those years, which will have tackled permanently this "powerful ghost'- 'money', helping to put 'money' back in the lower scale of our daily need preferences.

For centuries money have been causing: man to enslave others in the guise of - creating work for them to earn 'money'; man imprisoning himself in bondage for one life career out of fear of not having 'money'; man licking the dirty shoes of another in order to make money; man plotting the death of an innocent fellow for money sake; man taking a woman in marriage and vice versa, not out of love and affection for each other but for money'. People going through all the humiliations connected with prostitution; all for money. The list of the frustrating ventures and adventures which most humans go through on a daily basis for money's sake are innumerable.

HOW DO WE DESIGN A COMMON CURRENCY FOR ALL NATIONS?

The easiest way to do this will be to adopt one of the existing currencies or to design and print new currency as a global legal tender for all to use. The value of money is what it can buy, the satisfaction it can offer you, therefore, to accumulate wealth without deriving satisfaction out of it is worthless.

There is nothing wrong with having money or becoming a multimillionaire but, there is something wrong with it, when used in such a way that may cause trouble for others; particularly also, when money is placed above people, creativity and wisdom. People should be made to know that they cannot feed more than their stomach can contain; else, it will explode. This is another way to ask people to stop accumulating money and material wealth they may never be able to need. How many people in history had ever said "I do not want more; I have got enough; I am okay and contented with this which I have so far? Why are many not often using such phrases? Is it for the fear of the future or the fear of lack!

Let my people be taught to work enough to live and not to live to work- And to learn to lay most emphasis on creativity and selflessness than on money. Have respect and regards for other humans with or without-money.

In my view, I would rather opt for the old: **'BARTER-SYSTEM'**. The odds compared to the looming problems from the use of money as it is today will be more acceptable; or we could better unanimously adopt one of the most popular existing currencies such as: **Dollar, Pound Sterling or Euro to serve as our global legal-tender for all nations.** Also, I feel that money and material possession should henceforth, seize to be the yardstick with which to measure or determine the achievements of individuals or people; in its place- '*wisdom, degree or level of positive mental attitude (PMA) evidenced in a person's character trait (CCT), and amount or level of selfless services to others and environmental care will suffice*'. Such should become the basis for electing our true global icons; not money!

The above are sequence of things we can do, and ways we can reason in order to foster stability, peace, unity and harmony of this world as well as reduce crime, exodus, poverty and hunger!

RELIGION AND ITS PRACTICES

-One Religion for all Nations-

What is Religion?

A dictionary defines religion as: 'any of various systems of belief or worship concerned with the spiritual and inner nature of man and usually, a super natural power recognized as creator or controller.

From the look of things, religion occupies the third position in the category of things positively affecting and influencing mankind. But, lately the good and positive religious influences on people and society have taken a sharp down-turn; being diverted into very negative and mortal practice which is jarring everyone on the face and intruding in the form of belief chosen by others.

Truth is that the belief in something higher or extra-ordinary is a natural human characteristic; which best explains why we have these proliferations of religious organizations all across the wide world. In fact, there is nearly no one who does not have a belief in something; be it: Mysticism, shamanism up to- Hinduism, Buddhism, Taoism, Confucianism, Shinto, Judaism, Christianity, Apostasy, Islam etc.

It is obvious from these proliferations of beliefs in something supernatural that, religion as we have them today and from the past, is human invention to satisfy their natural crave for 'a good reason for this burden of living'.

Form of belief or religion should naturally be a personal affair, just like meditation, thinking and urinating are personal affairs; like all the rest of living matters: all the oceanic lives, all the jungle lives, all the underground lives, humans are as well created 'whole' to be very independent with a just supply of their basic needs as: food, water, shelter and clothing. Any other thing apart from those are nothing more than compliments and polishing of 'what there already was and still is'.

The good and bad Spirits silently living with you from the day you were born, should be the source of your belief; and your promises and decisions and choices you make with them pertaining the way you handle your daily and future affairs, should rightly be your business with them, and no one else's. God and Satan lives in you. They are your greatest teachers and your greatest ally, so what else are you searching for outside yourself that you do not have deep down within? The major principles and modes of conduct for peace and harmony for all mankind are boldly ingrained in the holy books; especially, 'the Bible' and 'the Koran'. They both embodies most of the universally-accepted moral standards meant for the purpose of attaining a closer and more intimate relationship with the Creator to whom all human species, tend to worship and glorify, whether consciously or otherwise. Through the demonstration of faith, hope and believe that the immediate future will always get better.

This is a way to encourage most people to be able to think positive and to do good while they await for their turn to toil, live and die and be jettisoned to the promised land where they will hopefully find-love, peace and harmony as their final reward for all these worldly hassles of being Alive!

Creed, faith in a particular system of belief or worship, democratically speaking, is supposed to be a private and personal affair. But, for which ever natural reason or of humanity; religious worship is no longer a matter of choice but of force and sometimes intimidation. And each day, there are alarming surge of men and women of God; most are real and most are false. Too much interpretation and re-interpretation of the original laws set down from the beginning meant to lead to salvation and maximum fulfillment for all human beings. To add or remove any part of those divine laws tantamount to sacrilege against the unseen and silent God or Creator! (Because doing so, tampering with things of creation obstructs the smooth processes of the affairs of life for millions of world citizens)

For these reasons and many more, the ex-IGPH students– ("special students trained to live and show effective, balanced lifestyle; also, global political reshuffle aimed to benefit every world citizen without partiality or favoritism") will have to review the entire global system of belief and worship in similar ways as for: Currency, Language and other important factors obstructing global peace, unity and harmony".

Nothing is absolutely impossible for humans to do if only they come together in unity with one idea pursuing it as a definite goal; surely, they must succeed to move further forward towards realizing whatever their collective or respective dreams may be".

Simple solution to all global religious problems

The ex-IGPH students are very much aware that there is no defined or given system of worship for the Creator. That the true consciousness of God or the Creator is all embedded deep within. The students or "the trained brand-new Leaders" will have to find a way to purify the religious sector from lots of false prophets, women and men of God proliferating that holy premises; finding an effective way to make it impossible for false prophets and false men and women of God delivering any form of deceptive and unfounded messages to the vulnerable public, who are innocently, simply seeking redemption and deliverance from the unknown.

I will suggest a uniform system of worship and belief for the entire human race- **from the look of things, all the religions and worships are focused on the same supreme being- one God and one Creator. So, why can't we all therefore worship one God under the same religious portfolio for unity and peace's sake?**

If all human races are able to worship the only Creator (if the Creator really needs to be worshipped) under one global religious platform; then we all will in turn benefit in the following ways: religious fanaticism will tend to decrease; Riots and killings connected to religion will also decrease. Xenophobia and religious intolerance will tend to decrease or cease outright. Terrorism and suicide bombing will decrease if not a total stop to it. Those minor problems are among the worst problems facing our past and modern times; helping us in nothing other than, tearing human races further apart from one another instead of bringing them nearer to each other.

-If humankind could be able to bring them to consciously practice and execute all of the above, things of this world shall certainly begin to improve to their possible best.

Otherwise, humanity as a whole will be busy singing Alleluia, clapping hands in praise of the lord, keeping night vigils in churches and at home, knocking and bashing their heads on stones and floors in prayers, starve themselves to death in prayers in the name of the unseen creator to no avail.

Trust me, my fellow humans!, Upon all that, you will still find yourselves millions of miles still far away from the promised land. Not only that, you will rather find yourselves retrogressing miles further away rather than miles further forward to this promised land as is everyone's ultimate desire!

Crime and violence will continue to multiply inflicting all mankind as stings of bees. Disease will be consuming you one by one in large numbers. Hunger and misery will painfully be sucking your blood and flesh like a pond leech.

Fear, terror and insecurity will dominate this world, keeping everyone scared and unsure of the next day if it comes and suffocates any trace of meaningful joy, peace unity and pleasure in our respective lives…

DRUG, ALCOHOL AND CIGARETTE

-Legalize them all or stop their Production Entirely-

So much have happened, so much is being said daily about drug, alcohol and cigarette. Obviously, the social issues involving the above items tend to be worsening in such an ascending progression; instead of decreasing progressively in proportion to the level of media publicities against them. Turn on your TV or Radio set anytime of the day, there must be one or more incidents about narcotic drugs. Most national and international publications- are talking about drugs, alcohol or dangers of cigarette every day.

On the other note:

People keep killing each other because of drug-issues; people caught and sent to prison because of drug; people constituting various social nuisances because of the effects of drug. On the other hand also, people of various age, hanging out in the city streets, some sleeping in bus and train stations for reasons connected to drugs or alcohol. Mortal road accidents caused by the negative effects of drugs and many more mishaps all directly or indirectly related to drug and alcohol'.

On other note, are the warnings and alarm raised by expert doctors on the dangers and imminent death posed by the constant use of alcohol, cigarettes and drugs etcetera.

"WARNING: CIGARETTE SMOKING IS DANGEROUS TO YOUR HEALTH" yet, its manufacturers keep making more attractive brands and propagandas aimed at selling more quantities and making more money. So, also, more and more youths tend to take more likeness to smoking than not, and to worsen this social problem the very use of those prohibited or partially prohibited items seem to be taking a dramatic increase; now lets talk about just drug.

WHAT IS DRUG?

A modern dictionary defines drug as: "a substance used in the treatment and prevention of sickness or disease; it is also defined as: a clinical substance, especially a narcotic, taken for the effect it produces".

Over the past four decades or so, much have being happening in relation to drug: many families (as in time of wars or national disasters) have been broken apart; many have lost their dear lives caused by direct or indirect involvement with drugs and others. Many people (especially the youth) have being continuously in and out of jails, while a good number of people as you read this, are still languishing in prisons for a long period of time for various laughable reasons; but, all tend to point accusing fingers to drug- its use, sale, manufacture and production.

GENERAL OVERVIEW

All of the above taken into consideration; it becomes relevant to add that this monstrous drugs form part of the things of creation and therefore, they are as old as mankind and their history. Although, the main emphasis lies on such metropolitan drugs such as: cocaine, ecstasy, heroine LSD, Marijuana, Hashish etcetera.

However, the fact that those drugs existed and happens to be addictive by their selves should not have constituted any kind of problem for any one. Because, also, there are various types of poisonous substances growing out there as drugs yet, their benefit to mankind when properly applied can also be many. The addictiveness of those drugs as cocaine, heroin are not the major problem but, rather, that aspect of human characteristics that when not disciplined, tends to push one towards over indulgence, which leads always to a voluntary or involuntary abuse of things of pleasure.

This is to say that, there is nothing created by the Creator that can be so harmful on its own if used and applied correctly. Even the food we accept and eat for sustenance, when wrongly eaten or abused, could also constitute an equal amount of disaster or ruin to an individual comfort and well being.

Knowing the long history of humankind never had anything being realized by human race without working them out by themselves. Humankind had always had problems with their- emotions, the food that they eat, the water that they drink, the air that they breathe, the child that they bear, and etcetera.

Your individual lives are in your hands; it's a fact of life. It is our respective duties as humans to manage our lives to achieve a sound and disciplined living style. Things are meant to revolve, revive and die. Everyone reasons, reacts and shows involuntary feelings in response to their given internal and external organ stimulus. Isn't it all part of the freedom of expression? All humans should listen and rely on their individual or collective efforts to control, moderate and discipline their needs and desires in conformity with the cosmic laws of the nature of things of creation. This is a compulsory global duty of every world citizen. Our global problems and challenges are not just drugs, alcohol or cigarettes, but, our wrong political values and dispensation of man-made things.

Therefore, the uses of narcotic drugs, cigarettes and alcohol are easily controllable as hard as it may sound; but, notwithstanding, it all boils down to 'the mental attitude' or the chemistry of mind-set and intrinsic values of the individual when it comes to the moments of "decision-making and action-taking".

Shakespeare visualized some of those human situations when he said: "our problems are not in our stars but in ourselves". Meaning that, nothing is beyond our control or management if we are sincerely willing to control and manage our given situations with caution and precaution; because, nothing under creation is a lone problem without causes and its ensuing effects!

WHAT SHOULD BE THE BEST PRACTICAL AND REALISTIC SOLUTION TO DRUG ISSUES CONSTANTLY MENACING OUR GLOBAL COMMUNITIES?

In order to really put an end to the present drug issues and their recurring social hazards spreading like epidemic in all nooks and corners of the world today; there are good reasons to suggest that- **"DRUGS, AS ALCOHOL AND CIGARETTES BE LEGALIZED"-**

-There is no way we can terminate the production and manufacture of drugs, for being one of the things of creation and fortunately or unfortunately, remedy for most of our bodily ailments when appropriately used and applied. -Such drugs in context induce euphoria and encourage intimate social relationships.

-The main advantage in legalizing drug usage will be to minimize this wanton break- up of families by the unforeseeable problems inherent in the use, sale, traffic and production of those narcotics.

-Legalizing those prohibited drugs will no doubt help to minimize the present recurring currency blockade and may bring peace and a new face-lift for many countries of the world marked 'RED' on global maps; such countries as: Central America (Columbia), Afghanistan and many others.

-Legalization of those prohibited drugs will help to minimize the unnecessary and indiscriminate congestions of prisons, wastage of manpower from the part of unproductive people forced to live in jail for so long and the waste of constructing and maintaining new prisons and their inmates.

-Above all, the legalization of those drugs will help to make them unattractive for those people who seek for quick avenues to get rich; or make a decent living without much sweat.

-That will also help to bring back most of our talented youth who are being led astray through that monstrous and unproductive world of drug, delinquency and prison.

-If possible, let our respectable news media desist from giving constant and daily attention to those narcotic drugs- such approach is in no way positive. Because in compliance with natural human psychology; such approach to the deeper problem of drug can only help to attract more people going after drug because it is in vogue; it is always on the news; this is normal and common human characteristics. We all want to go with the latest on the news, with what is in vogue!

To achieve the above, the ex-IGPH- will have to devise an appropriate means and strategy to legalize the sale, use and dispensation of said drugs or narcotics.

LICENSING, SALE AND DISPENSATION

-After legalizing the use and possession of those drugs in context, the licensing and dispensation have to be worked out by a global consensus. Every nation should be part of this and should be able to open their mind to this new era of things; let's give this a sincere try at least, to watch and see how this system will get better for all humans.

-We should work out the modalities to manufacture and package the narcotics in well controlled and safe doses; in a similar way as we do with many other dangerous drugs that are being prescribed by experts in the field.

-They can either be acquired or obtained by prescription or be allowed to be in a free market as alcohol and cigarettes. Or rather, let drugs be dispensed in pharmaceutical shops; or set up a brand new organization which will be specifically made in charge of all matters concerning narcotic drugs: its manufacture, dispatching, sale and usage. To manage also, all monies realized from all transactions in connection to any drug's dispensed and distributed to the final consumers.

-There is no doubt that this simple measure will surely help to sabotage the exorbitant drug prices, which is pushing many youths into robbery and anti-social behaviors as evidenced everywhere today in all over our global communities.

-The simple logic here is- If narcotics cease to be a "quick-money-maker" putting into considerations all human tendencies, desires and natural reactions to things and situations- those people who are presently being favorably dependent on its easy money will naturally have to begin to search for other avenues to "get-rich- quick".

-This will also help to ease and relax the daily news features on drugs.

-Most families torn apart by drug related offenses will be reunited.

-Prisons will be decongested; lots of money and manpower will be saved and put into more lucrative activities beneficial to the general public.

-Above all, the majority of our youths, (our future leaders) already being led astray, and, who are presently living in limbo, will be recovered through legalizing the use of that 'monstrous drug'. This kind of moves by our global leaders will conform to this new era of changes which will aim to foster; in these ways we can have the unbridled chance to global peace, unity and harmony under total equality. "YES WE CAN"!

WEAPONS AND ARMED FORCES

Weapons are devices or instruments meticulously fabricated with the final aim to fight, immobilize or instantly kill animals and even human beings. If the weapons are in metallic form, they possess the capacity to also demolish houses and buildings. When composed of liquid substances can demolish an entire ecosystem: plants, insects and animals of all categories.

The big question remains as thus: **That if weapons are meant to destroy and take away precious lives of fellow men and women, destroy houses and precious works of arts, what is therefore the essence of its constant fabrication and proliferation?**

Yes, certain period in human history, out of ignorance, it was deemed normal or even very necessary to have the best weapon to defend oneself and family; the sovereignty or the country of one's own origin. Then, it was a trendy attitude and universally accepted as normal. But, we as a unique human race have come a very long way these days with a higher level of intelligence more than enough to know and understand the importance of: love, peace, unity and harmony to our good health and that of our environment in their entirety.

The universe as a whole has been converted to a small community because of technological advancement; more integration, more unity with nearly everyone speaking the same language as brothers and sisters; who we really are, in the sight of the Creator. Reasoning in this line of thought, it becomes obvious that the present obsessive attitude of all nations to willingly proliferate weapons of mass destruction is in no way the best move or approach closer to realizing that profound universal desire and quest for peace, unity and harmony at all levels!

But, in order to restore discipline and viable laws to control this 'war-zone', the ex-IGPH will have to devise ways to harness all weapons of mass destruction from every nation and use them to set up a "World Class Museum", where people from other planets can visit and appreciate our human ingenuity and prowess in our technological advancement. All the weapons can also be assembled for the general public to visit and see what their fellow humans have achieved in all those years.

If there is: peace, love and unity amongst humans, will there be any more need for those destructive armaments?

As entire mankind will soon be united in love and oneness, there is going to be no more need for such instruments of warfare and destruction. There will be no more territories to defend because will make our boarders open and become free for all humankind to go in and to come out at will.

DO HUMANS HAVE NATURAL NEED FOR WEAPONS?

The answer is a capital "YES"! But, not weapons of mass destruction; small and personal weapons of safe defense; "yes"!

If true that "the destiny of humankind is in their hands", so should be their physical defense; in their hands as well'. This into perspective, therefore, it will be advisable to legalize a short pistol of only two rounds for every adult; and the present hunting guns can still remain in use as of now. And also be legalized for the purposes of hunting and ceremonies in which gun shots may be required.

Every man and woman has a need for self defense. Naturally, it is not wise for a human being to walk around unprotected by any form of instrument or weapon. Our world had always been a jungle where the fittest wants to live and feed on the weak. Sometimes, it could be a member of your family who loses mental equilibrium and tends to eliminate an entire family with a gun or other deadly weapon; maybe, for being the only one in that family who is in possession of a gun or other weapon at that moment of disequilibrium. Who can stop such a person from wiping out a whole family if such a situation occurs? Because, most of the times, in situations like these, before the arrival of relevant authorities to such scenes- usually the damage is already done!

Sometimes also, it could happen that your pet animal, such as your dog or any other domestic animal may get wild and attacks its owner or any other member of the family or neighborhood, what could you do to save the situation at that moment? These things happen nearly on daily bases in different parts of the world at a given moment in time; and whenever they do happen, we should see them as normal life occurrences.

Nevertheless, our human duty should be to prepare ourselves and try to prevent major excesses when they occur. Therefore, it is my view that, outright prohibition of anything is wrong; and runs against the nature of the free human will and adventure. Outright prohibition of anything does not portray a cautious and proactive system strategy. Unless there are other ulterior motives that made past and incumbent systems to place such outright bans on things as weapons, drug, etc. Or is it better for the general public not to know the real aims of the laws supposed to lead them towards the protocol of: love, peace, unity and harmony?!

Assume we accept the above suggestions, the ex-IGPH will have to set up a global body responsible for: manufacture, licensing, control and distribution of any firearm released in the market through licensed and authorized dealers.

Initially, it will be pertinent to start this operation with 'gum bullets' capable only to immobilize an enemy for two to three hours, which should be enough time before help comes to someone in a situation of attack or danger. You do not necessarily need to kill to bring or maintain peace. The hunter's gun can be maintained as it is or modified to suit the present situation of things.

Then, all the warships, warplanes, missiles and other mass destruction weapons should be made to be assembled either, in a chosen place or manned by a special body in each country wherever such destructive weapons may be located. (This should better be left to the discretion of the competent appointed body) those weapons as monstrous as they may be, in some degree, portrays and represents one of the highest levels of human ingenuity and technological advancement. And therefore, be treated with adoration. Our Arms depot and most military barracks should be converted into areas for tourist attractions for Earth citizens and for the people visiting the Earth from outer space.

Having done all that, the great men and women of wars (all the Armed Forces) should be set free and released from the camps and barracks, to go back to their respective homes; to catch some rest with families and begin to pursue their personal goals in life. If any may wish to divert into other fields wherever their disciplined services may be required for the benefit of many others that will be fine enough.

Better still, the majority of the soldiers should be organized to combine their united combat discipline in a united effort to battle and overcome food shortages, hunger and diseases through a unified global farming system and disease eradication techniques.

The level of mental and physical discipline of a soldier, applied conscientiously in any field of activity will never fail to yield fruit. The soldiers have got all it takes to set the engine of successful change churning. I suggest we should capitalize on their expertise to save both people and animal lives only; and not to take any life away.

In a similar way, the ex-IGPH students will have to sit back and meticulously scrutinize most of the big organizations with many followers such as: sports and religious organizations; find a way to utilize most of their combined human power or workforce to render more practical assistance to the governing body in the field of **farming and eradication of hunger and diseases.** Most men and women of God should or will have to team up with the military experts and device a functional method to produce and provide food in abundance and maybe, also shelter for the general populace.

Because the road to the 'Promised Land' is very far away-hunger and lack of adequate rest and stress surely reduces people's chances by over one thousand percent far from reaching their respective destinations'

It is visualized that, if mankind could convert all or most of their energy, expertise and ingenuity which are negatively being invested into fighting and killing; and arms manufacture and proliferation, the global citizens will have enough to eat and drink if duly harnessed. And if, also our global leaders could be able to design a way to invest most human energies into positive ventures; for example, in the areas of farming and reconstruction, there should be food and drink for the entire global citizens to feast. And also harnessing the abundant amount of energy spent on global perspectives, in daily basis by all men and women of God, which they spend for worshipping; preaching and praying day-in day-out, in hope for celestial miracles; harnessing such combined energy and talent into agricultural research and food production and manufacture, I will stake anything that, the entire humans race, their plants and animals will definitely have enough to eat and to drink forever, for so long and there shall be no more lack of food, water and merriment for the entire humanity and the ecosystem in general!

People will be more merry and happy with their stomach full. They will be more enthusiastic about most of things of creation and the entire world will benefit more in a system replete with more enthusiastic generation.

All of the above may not bring a lasting solution to most of the present global problems but, at least, we will be embarking on a possible major solution. You are being sincere in your search for a lasting solution to the problems overwhelming your global order. This is what counts most between man and God; doing your best and leaving the rest to God the Creator!

Confident enough that, if humanity could adopt the above initiative – I promise, in a space of only ten years after the adoption, every human will cease to worry about what to eat and where to sleep or what to wear; trust me! The veritable sense of unity and equality will definitely ensure for all humanity!

THE POLICE FORCE

The Police literally means: law enforcement agent; organized forces of men and women trained to harness their energy with a uniform discipline of purpose; and with an aim to enforce and maintain the current laws of each government wherever and whichever they are assigned to represent, for the smooth and harmonious dispensation of law and justice for the benefit of the people of that given region or country.

In the present order of things, the entire police forces will have to be reshuffled in order to embrace this new concept of re-channeling the affairs of this world to the betterment of entire humanity. And to do all that and give credence to this new concept- police

-All the activities of the police will have to be controlled and directed by one central body which will be set-up by the ex-IGPH students.

-The police forces will have to be retrained to quench riots of various dimensions and acts of indiscipline and vandalism without the use of mortal weapons. And if they have to carry and use any weapon at all, it has to be weapons that are capable only to immobilize culprits for a couple of hours without killing or doing serious damage or harm to them.

-Each region or nation will have to continue to enjoy the protection and services of indigenous men and women under the system name- **'community-policing'** which will be managed and controlled through the mandate of a **Global Police Headquarters**. We cannot rely on the hope that everyone will consciously do things right, but, however, we strongly hope that these policies must help to mitigate the majority of the negative conducts streaming in the veins of a good number of humankind.

-The police will be given the responsibility to keep vigilance and to police all the rest of the governmental organs; including the general public. They will police the incumbent leaders, the public, the finance, schools, religious bodies and the department of justice etcetera. And also to persuade that everyone keep and obey those laws and orders with a reasonable deep sense of patriotism.

-Offenders who fall under this new system of things will have to face not an arbitrary judge or judgment; but, a kind of judgment dispensed by the community members themselves; who will be elected through unanimous decision. They shall be bestowed with the powers to represent and reflect the common feelings of the given community where the said offense must have taken place and what made the offender to have committed the said crime or wrongdoing.

WHAT TYPE OF JUDICIAL SYSTEM WILL BE MOST APPROPRIATE FOR THIS NEW ERA OF THINGS AND CAN ALSO RELIEF THE HEAVY SECURITY BURDEN ON POLICE FORCES?

I will suggest for a judicial system similar to that of the 'Crown Court' as is being practiced in the UK. Each regional community will have only one or two Crown Courts depending on size of the region and inhabitants. Every 'Crown Court' will have to be presided over by a local legal representative appointed from the 'global judicial headquarters'. The global judicial headquarters will be solely responsible to make a final decision upon all global judicial affairs such as: appointing the 'Crown Court' judges, hearing of all Appeal cases, and establishment of 'Crown Courts' wherever due and necessary etc. And whose other job will be to seal, either way, the decisions of the jury members.

Some minor offenses should be allowed to be resolved and dealt with at the local jury levels; but, some serious cases that may hamper mass peace and tranquility should have to be forwarded to the notice of the central headquarters for appropriate deliberation. Justice has to be allowed to proceed smoothly without fear or favor. It should always aim to ascertain that no single individual be victimized in any given circumstances.

-Every case should be carefully listened to, examined without bias or prejudice; and not only basing judgments on face values or on the horrors of an offense committed; the best approach to justice is to lay more emphasis on the reasons and motives behind every offense- It is most natural for people to react over matters affecting them according to their personal convictions and impulses. Therefore, in any given case or breach of the laws in a community or nation, the members of the jury should always try to feel themselves in the shoes of the offender. Doing so will help them more to understand the ulterior motive of that culprit being accused; if his or her reaction to the committed offense should be viewed and considered, as a natural human reaction basing on what provoked the individual to such a crime. To preach and bring honest justice in any human system of government, the judges must take into account how they as judges and other public may react if they find themselves in the situation the culprit standing judgment before them will react if confronted or found in a similar situation. That is 'the-must-have' spirit of true justice.

-If found that the motive for the offense be based on intentional aggravation or self-defense, the culprit will be allowed to go home or given the most minimum sentence possible irrespective of the gravity of the offense committed- that is the aim of justice; and never to take these things too personally.

-Such offenses without enough evidences, the accused should usually be given the benefit of the doubt; case dismissed and the defendant be admonished and pleaded with to sin no more.

-The community or state should never try to condemn any one when the offense is not beyond reasonable doubt. All the global human communities should be sensitized and made to know that their security and their judicial balance are in their respective hands and should as a matter of patriotism, always report, any act of indiscipline or misconduct to the appropriate body or police in charge of that region.

-It is not nice that people should let things around them to go wrong and wait for the government or police to figure things out by themselves alone. The system is for all and never for those in power alone. If everyone helps to control crime and fight injustice and indiscipline, things will surely function a lot better for all.

-If the global community is able to fight and reduce or eliminate crime out of their collective and individual volition or participation, then, the rest of the lawyers will have no more need to their present jobs and therefore, can go into other sectors or more lucrative businesses of their choice or try to convert their collective talents into other sectors of public services more profitable to humanity; same thing for the prison workers etcetera!

-Imagine the amount of money and manpower to be saved and better utilized for agricultural researches and food production if we are able to peacefully do away with prisons and criminal lawyers; in a situation where peace, love and harmony should reign supreme in our global communities! All the criminal lawyers, prison warders and prison inmates voluntarily becoming food producers and caretakers of things of creation! How I wish to live to see that day come true!

-However, the ex-IGPH students will find a better way to harness these delicate issues for all to benefit mutually and amicably.

TAXES AND TAXATION

-NO MORE TAXES ON PEOPLE'S ACTIVITIES OR PROPERTIES-

Taxes; for whatever purpose they may serve or have been serving till now, should have to be stopped. There should be no more taxes of any kind, whether from individuals, companies, organizations or properties. People should be encouraged to work freely, learn freely and manage freely the wages of their sweat without any form of intrusion.

-Whenever the government needs money for any form of project should have to make that amount from any of the numerous natural resources endowed upon the world by the Creator. Out of that, they (the governing body) should have to pay salaries, create jobs and save for projects intended for social development.

-Taxation on people's efforts and proceeds have the uncanny feel and connotation of oppression and suppression- anything that had to be done by force and with coercion never make happy anyone – such ugly feelings are against the spirit of this new order of things! Taking money from the 'have-nots' does not make any good impressions whatsoever; irrespective of how genuine your reasons could be.

-It is very ugly when mentors, teachers or guardians who are supposed to cater and nurture their supposed children, start asking – rather forcing their children: to pay money to them as TAX because they work; to pay because they feed, to pay because they live in a house or to pay because their vehicles apply tarred roads which were naturally meant for all to use; etcetera.

The act of taxation on the general public, seen from the humane point of view of the order of natural things within creation, gives the same ugly impression like of those abusive parents who intentionally send their young and fragile children out to the street to work and beg for alms while they stay home: eating, drinking, merriment and waiting for their children to return with food and money to support their parental self aggrandizement at the very expense of their weak and fragile children. For this very reason and many more, taxation has to be deleted from our world lexicon!

What should replace direct and indirect taxes?

-In place of direct taxes on people and properties, the ex-IGPH students will have to set up a central global body with representatives in all over the regions of every nation, who shall be fully in charge of collecting regular voluntary donations from the general public. They can apply the same tactics used by the religious organizations if they are unable to devise a better way to get assistance from the global public; also the national populace should be sensitized on the regular need to or whenever possible, as a matter of national duty, contribute to the established global organization.

-The said organization in return, will be responsible for sponsoring all government and public projects; sponsor also, individual talents and ideas that shall benefit the general public when accomplished.

-The said organization should better collaborate with all the banking institutions for loaning money and financial assistance to the general public that are genuinely in need of the money and with a viable project that will pay back the loan without interest or with a token of interest rate.

-The banking industry will have to be reviewed- in fact, the bankers themselves should have to come together and find other ways to encourage people to manage their money in a way that using cash and liquid money be discouraged; also to make it that robbers and bums, be discouraged from thinking and seeing the banking industry as a gateway to quick and easy source of money.

My piece of advice:

-Fervently living and following the natural laws of creation at all times and in all things, I found out that, people will most voluntarily give away nearly all they own to support a just cause; be it national or personal cause, than when they are reminded or forced to give their hard-earned effort away over shady causes. This is going to be the new global spiritual attitude towards all things concerning humankind; doing good deeds at will.

-We should try to give and rely on the day to day running of the affairs of the society to the: police, the community jury, the funding organizations and above all to the genuine News Media organizations.

-I will suggest that the News Media should be allowed complete freedom of expression. They are or should be the **'global eyes'** working hand-in-hand with the police force; and with this, globalize the news media world and stop the present system of selling information meant to educate or enlighten the general public.

-People should be made to stop buying and selling information; education and information should be as free as the air that we breathe.

-This is because, the ultimate pleasure derivable from or out of any experience or acquired knowledge is only in the **act of sharing** them with others and that is what we intend to try to do in this present order of things. The news media and the police have to be paid and sponsored by the funding body.

-The global news media should always offer: free services, completely free and fair information, and globalized information dissemination!

SCHOOL AND SCHOOLING

-SELF-EDUCATION SHOULD BE PARAMOUNT FOR ALL-

The main aim for school and schooling is certainly for easy and synchronized indoctrination of the general public for the benefit of all through: mutual communication and global collaboration!

School is an institution of learning where different subjects are being taught and imparted at various levels, for the main purpose of making as many people as possible to know the same thing, think in the same way; so that they can uniformly apply the acquired discipline or knowledge whenever and wherever the need may arise within the periphery of our collective global community; be it within the far future or in the immediate present.

There are lots of essential activities necessary to give the best possible education to our beloved children without sending them away from the comforts of their homes:

1. Stop sending your children to *schools* under coercion or obligation to obey and serve a faceless academic

institution which does not teach our children how to achieve self sufficiency, independence and how to positively manage and balance their given lives!

2. As a parent, it is your natural duty to educate your children the best way possible apart from feeding them and paying for their respective social needs.

3. As a parent you must, as a natural obligation positively impart to your children in accord to your inherited, acquired or discovered knowledge of life leading to the positive pathway of living.

4. As a parent, it is your natural duty to teach your given children how to: think and act positive, how to play positive, how to positively deal with most affairs of life according to what you know growing up before becoming a parent today.

5. Above all, you must as a parent teach your beloved child/children how to do the basic and fundamental things of life such as cooking and balanced eating habits, hygiene and home caring, how to produce food and care for plants and animals which they cannot live without; how to embrace the natural sense of self-initiative which happens to be the basic rule for attaining self education. Self education is in all essence the only and most valid form of learning which in every human can restore balance and indelible knowledge!

6. If everyone's personal talents are different as our finger-prints, how then can a generalized academic knowledge teach a child to discover his or her given natural potentials and use it for good?

7. -Every parent should be allowed the sole right to train

their hard earned children in their own ways; at least give them a seventy percent time to impart whatever they have in them to their children; and education given by institutions should be free and non-obligatory.

8. -It is a gross crime against creation and humanity in a broader sense to prevent a living being not to think, talk and act freely out of his or her own given mind. Without the due expression of the inner thought from an individual, how on earth can we know the natural inclination and possible personality of an individual?

9. -How can you claim to be well educated and learned without due and adequate time to yourself invested in meditation for innermost thought and scrutiny prior to personal views and conclusions? What then is the rightful job of the magnificent human brain; the eyes, the ears and the sense organs? Are those no more the natural given organs for any sane individual to learn and to know at will whatsoever he or she wishes or strives to know if let alone or assisted accordingly?

The above views into consideration, the ex-IGPH students will have to review the entire academic systems for the kind of subjects being imparted to children and adults as well; and classify them according to their level of importance or benefit to the combined society of humankind.

-Subjects such as: biology, chemistry, physics, mathematics, geography etcetera with universal formulae should be allowed to continue to be taught in schools to at least a basic level, because they bear laws and formulae that have been helpful to humankind to bind things of imagination and creation together since time immemorial; for the enhancement of technological and social advancement.

-The rest of the subjects should or can be made optional. People should be made to study at leisure and in harmony with their natural potentials avoiding any kind of obligation on any subject matter.

-Subjects such as: Religion, history, sociology archaeology etcetera, are alright to be made optional as school or academic subjects; in order to keep such subjects alive, not because they are that important or necessary for our wellbeing. They should be encouraged through documentaries, movies, televisions and computer programs for everyone to see and know; especially, for the children to know a bit of past history.

-Work and rewards should be based on individual abilities, determination and willingness to work and learn to do a given job without putting into consideration the level of education or studies carried out or attained. I see it more appropriate to reward the level of experience, dedication to a particular profession or job than the level of academic education acquired. People should avoid being in a hurry to do or finish a given job, attain fame and to make money or material aggrandizement; it is more rewarding instead, to aim to do your respective best and to do most of the things which you engage fully well and correctly.

-Education or academic studies are in the same category as physical exercises and games; they are both personal initiatives to better one through doing something which one is talented in or passionate about, therefore, should be free for all to benefit.

-I feel that the level of education or time spent studying a particular subject at school, as well as political engagements should not be the basis for economic rewards; it is much better if we can begin to encourage and reward the real work done or output in positive services to others.

-Teachers, media men and women, authors and writers of various categories should be paid, pampered for their respective contributions in educating and disseminating information that helps to motivate the general public towards sound and good behaviors which promotes global peace and harmony. Meaning to say that, we should begin henceforth to reward the positive contributions as a way to encourage more people doing good services to others, instead of rewarding academic or school attendances of people and the amount of certificates they accumulated.

-Schools, schooling and academic education are good attributes to acquire; but, please let every human know that, true education is a personal decision or that in which one is encouraged by relatives to engage upon.

That the best educated people are not those who went through the academic walls; but, those who know where and how to get whatever they need to realize their set-goals in life; and in harmony without violating anyone else's right. We go to school because we feel it's best; in the same way we can do very well without school if all things be allowed to remain equal.

-Enough of these peoples' indoctrination and suppression of their natural intelligence! Let people think and reason out things for themselves so that, in these ways, respect and family have a better chance to be close to each other once again as it used to be in the past before all these phantasmagoric institutions sprang up out of the thin air through some wicket legislations that are intended to divide and rule than unify and bind.

-Today, with the presence of computers and internet, more than ever before, it is just enough to employ them to teach our children at the comfort of their homes to learn to read and write just for the sole purpose of social communication, cohesion and integration. While they are busy learning to read and write, we will be accessing them to discover their real and natural potential inclination. Yes! These are some of the best ways to begin to regain our natural aptitude for learning and expression of thoughts and instincts. I bet you, in these ways, every child will be more cheerful, more clever, more useful to themselves, their families and ultimately to their respective societies at large.

-When any child is allowed or duly directed to make use of their natural talents in what they have the flare for it, yes, learning for that very child will become fun and in few years, in less than two to three years doing that, they will begin to produce phenomenal and exceptional results. This is the true nature of humans as specie.

-No one is comfortable spending all those donkey years in an established institution of brain-wash called schools and so forth. That should be over now by this mandate. Our schools are producing so many depressed kids, beggars, aloof people and, indifference and nonchalant and above all delinquents and utter unproductive humans. Basta ya! Enough!

WORK AND WORKING

-FIVE-HOUR WORK DAILY FOR ALL GLOBAL CITIZENS-

- Work and working from today, in this new era of things should be accepted and designed as **'labor of love and joy'** we must be able to work for the most, to benefit others and so should others work to benefit you yourself; this way is sharing, and sharing multiplies earnings and also carries to everyone- love and happiness; that is one of nature's laws. The more you are able to give in service to others, the most you receive in reward: physically, spiritually and materially. Do not underestimate these principles of life!

- All work in this world had been long completed and done-with by the Creator; every human should always bear in mind that, they have got no job anymore left for them to do on earth to help in creating any new thing. Your only work is to live-out your lives with the things of nature within your vicinity; the rest of the things you may import or refine are compliments and cosmetics. Like your: dog, horse, chicken or even the fly lives out their nature in calm, peace and harmony wherever they find themselves at any given moment in time; but humans always want to recreate out of that which had been created; fantasize and analyze things which they see or hear; humans being among the weakest and feeblest of all the creatures are constantly driven by fear of death; for which they spend their entire earth life in search of security through: food, clothe, house or shade. This is just pure human nature; there is nothing wrong with our human nature. Man, like all other creatures are created to survive independent of any external assistance other than natural materials provided to them within the vicinity of their respective habitat.

-Working yourself to exhaustion is a sign of ignorance, fear and frustration; don't you see that in your entire bid to make your lives and the world better as you say, you are only working against the wind; as a result, you are obstructing the natural course of things of creation. It is all vanity at the end of the road which you must meet on the long run.

- Do not take yourselves very seriously because your life and the act of living are meant to be a thing of pleasure and not that of war and just fruitless laboring.

-Try to give much time to yourself in meditation, contemplation, appreciation and physical and mental exercises; the remaining of your time should be shared between the joyful works you dedicate to do, and the people around you; with nature as your medium or energy source. This is living with nature as a creature and not as the Creator.

-Share and enjoy each other and not use and hate each other; this is negative living that gives no better reward.

-Work is the act of expending one's energy to realize a synchronized activity with the aim to achieve economic, material or spiritual benefit for the growth and betterment of oneself, others and the things of creation within the entire eco-system.

-Working is a necessary exercise or ingredient of nature for the purpose of refurbishing and fortifying the degenerative tissues of human muscles and organs meant to regularly maintain a sound and healthy body. For this, all forms of work should be felt as a medium to pleasure; contrarily, any act or work that fails to give or provide pleasurable conditions, is not good enough for you and should not be continued for long.

-Whenever you may engage upon any job or work that does not accrue a pleasurable sensation; the time given to that working hours is wasted due to the fact that the inherent pleasure of doing a thing is in that moment being denied. Work in that moment becomes a source of torture instead of a source of pleasure.

-But on the contrary, when we do or engage upon works that we like and enjoy doing, this triggers a pleasurable sensation which aids psychological and physical healthiness which also, usually motivates one to give one's very best; and this situation or state of mind, is the basis and essence of all human achievements in the field of work and sound mental imagination.

-That is the main spirit behind all the wonders ever performed by humankind in the world you and I today live in. All that we see and assume as technology and great works of art are based on works of passion executed by people motivated either out of difficulties or inspirations, beliefs and faith in the things they do. Therefore, lets learn to do works that we like and enjoy doing; let's try to employ people in the works that they show natural inclinations, or penchant toward them and avoid doing work just for the money and material benefits we can get off them – that is the main source of depression and unhappiness which is more common nowadays in places of work; and why most people are daily yielding less and less of their natural potentials every day that passes!

-Each time anyone starts a business, whether funded by the funding body or not, if that person chooses to hire extra work force as done by companies or big businesses- in such cases, the employees or workers should be paid by the employer n collaboration with the central funding body; who in turn will have to pay those workers according to the existing service norms. People will no more be paid salaries by employers, their service salaries should come through the centralized funding body; this will enhance fairness and cutoff abuses.

-The business owners should pay themselves with the money they are making from their businesses and owe no allegiance whatsoever, to no one specifically. The only obligation being that business owners should once in a while give a regular tithe or donations to the Funding body' which they should honestly use for projects aimed at social and technological development.

-This new system of things should encourage the majority of global citizens to work more for themselves at their own comfortable times of the day or night without limitations and obligations of any type whatsoever. This is the only justifiable way to make majority of global citizens to inculcate the good habit of going the extra-mile at all times and in every form of work or activities they may be engaged with.

-Is there any working adult who do not know the agony of going to work for a boss; or the joy of working for oneself at one's own schedule? The fact is that whenever we work for ourselves, especially in activities we like, we tend to work for much more time and render much more fruit; for this very reason we want to change most of that old working conditions to make work for every global citizen, a thing of joy instead of a thing of torture and constant agony, given that, we must have to spend our entire lifetime doing just that- working.

-It's a rule of nature; the moment you stop working hard and happy, that very moment you start to die and atrophy without knowing it! All the money and material wealth cannot save you or reverse that nature's law; as it is for the wretched and poor to sick and die, so also it is for the rich and wealthy. No one can escape physical and mental exercises or challenges for long and remain so healthy both the poor and the rich! So love your work please, and learn to work with joy and enthusiasm for serenity sake!

RETIREMENT SCHEME

-NO MORE RETIREMENT FOR ALL GLOBAL CITIZENS-

What is retirement?

Retirement is withdrawal from active services; simply, to give up working!

The question is: what is the rationale or real meaning of retiring oneself or for someone to give up active work or services for oneself and to others?

What should a healthy person do if he/she should stop to work for himself or serve others? Sleep away the rest of their life time; embark on roaming aimlessly around the world in search of pleasure/adventure; or better still, live and rot in any small Island sunbathing as is generally accepted and practiced in these recent years?

Know it all that, our respective human minds as a rule of nature, feeds and grows better through effective usage and conversely atrophies and deteriorates without active and effective use!

For this very reason, for people to retire from active work or services for themselves and to others is, synonymous to spiritual death-warrant! Why? Because it is nature's rule that, each time you give, automatically you receive in proportion to that given on the spur of that moment; and, the moment you stop giving you also will seize to receive! The human mind is a natural organ that responds only to the specifics of nature's principles and cannot fully respond to human influences or manipulations; therefore, our human mind knows not the meaning of such things as: time, age, years, today, tomorrow worst still, retirement. You cannot carry over the joy, pleasure, or pain of this moment to another day or another moment. Human mind or spirit does not function with the tangibles but, with the intangibles; if it were to function well with riches and material possessions, I feel, almost all people in America and Europe should have been the happiest humans on earth; but, are they?

As I write this piece, I live not more than ten meters in front of the sea with my family in the South of Tenerife, in the Canary Island of Spain. I assure you, ninety percent of my neighbors are retired people from all parts of what you refer to as 'civilized world': Germans, British, Italians, Swedish, French etcetera. In reality, entire Canary Island is constructed and built as it is today, mostly for the money from these retirees and subventions from other sources.

Apart from those who come and go daily on vacation alone, majority of the inhabitants on this Island own their dream houses and live in absolute human comfort per se.

Irrespective of living in the supposed human comfort, what struck me most is seeing the highest degree of spiritual and physical deterioration amongst these retired people; most among them are invalids, others who are well are so wrinkled and worn-out that all the good food and money in this world can no more resuscitate and add more life to them!

I also know that, nearly all or most of these people had worked or served their nation in various fields for nothing less than thirty and forty years of their respective youthful lives; some have even worked for more time battling daily in snow and extreme weather conditions in hope and wait for these retirement days.

Understand that to live a good and balanced life, a reasonable amount of positive energy is required to be expended on a daily basis from you, without which money and all material possessions you may have accumulated are rendered worthless for health related issues which will confront you more often than not.

My grandfather died at hundred and five years (105yrs) he was already eighty-four years (84yrs) before my birth and I can assure you, as I write this at forty-nine having travelled, worked and lived in nearly all the continents of this world, I have never met people with the kind of energy and what I refer to as a good life; like my grandfather and those of his generation. My grandmother as well, was ninety eight (98) when she died. But, I can assure you that they never had: social security, never received pensions, never had doctors and nurses catering for them nor could they read or write; but, they still had everything in abundance from 'Mother-Nature' and lived a long and healthy live.

In such ages, my grandpa and grandma were used to walking on their barefoot, for over four-eight kilometers all day going to and from their vast farms to work and back home when they got tired. Every day, they usually eat well out of their produce and also rest very well; make fiestas, attend to community meetings, visit friends and be visited by friends.

They were always doing all their things with constant entertainment day and night. In the end, they always had excesses of everything both for themselves, family and for friends. I saw them constantly sharing food and all things amongst themselves with joy, unity and respect for each other, with "Mother Nature" and the culture that bind them together as a kindred or tribe.

Certainly, I have never seen or lived such peace and harmony ever since I left that environment and that generation!

It's a big shame and disappointment upon all our civilizations and development that, we are in this present generation unable to achieve such level of unity, peace and harmony amongst ourselves. Those days were the only period of my life I witnessed brotherhood and sisterhood in all neighborhoods. And, I must confess that still hold to highest esteem the decades during the lives of my grandparents; in that period, I learnt some things that I really enjoyed and managed to retain till today. The only aspect of that past which I do not fully accept were their numerous superstitions.

The best thing done by our ancestors in their days was their sustained adherence in harmony and respect to Mother Nature; they flowed with the tide instead of going against it as we do today in all our frenetic and uncontrolled efforts to negatively and forcefully challenge and work against our 'Beloved Mother Nature'.

RECOMMENDATION

-Considering the huge benefit of work for the human mind and body, in that context, I will suggest that we should allow people to work or give their services to themselves and to their respective communities willingly as far as, and in as much as they are able to without hindrances or obligations of any kind whatsoever!

-We should employ people only in jobs they like to do, especially those in which we notice that they have got a natural talent for them.

-instead of retiring our advanced and experienced workers, we should best form a global association for ex-workers of every field of work who will continue to impart and impact their years of experiences on the growing youths better than rendering them and their years of experiences null and void; this way they will continue to feel useful and helpful for their growing youth and to our society in general. That will as well encourage their mind to continue to give and receive than to reduce them only to the receiving end.

-No matter how little anyone's mind is able to function, if that mind is connected to the cord of positive mental attitude, as physically handicapped that person may happen to be, can still do big things and achieve awesome results which could benefit that person and others in no small measures.

-we should stop making life easy for ourselves without minimum struggles or efforts, because, doing so is utterly inimical to sound health and good living on the long run.

-We should learn to face old age without fear and worry and accept it instead with tranquility and as natural as part of the processes of life and living, period.

-No need to panic and fret about what happens to us at old age and when we are sick; what you fear most comes to you sooner or later as nature's rule; Stop worrying, never stop doing things and keeping your mind and hands as busy as you can afford to; be happy and plan better because that's all you actually owe to yourself, the world and to the Creator and let what will be to be; period!

CELEBRATIONS AND FIESTAS

-COMPULSORY CELEBRATION DAYS FOR ALL CITIZENS-

Celebrations and fiestas are the best aspect of all human existence. It is the only human feeling that cannot be faked, that breaks all barriers, permits no limitations for genders, creed or origin. It is the most encompassing human feeling of all time; the best positive human endowment which unites one with oneself, others and the unseen spirits. Celebrations are wholesome food for the souls of every living and non-living organs. Fiestas are a lubricant to the human bones and joints, body builder and brain cleanser…so let's celebrate at all moments!

We have to start to celebrate every day that we are alive to rekindle the sunlight in us at   all moments. Such feelings or emotions should be every day; we should map out moments of celebrations or fiestas every day as we do with all other things, don't you agree?

We should endeavor to stop that tendency to suffocate our good feelings to being happy and enjoying our lives to the fullest. What sense does it make to wait to celebrate Christmas, New Years, and birthdays and all such while we should rightly celebrate every moment of our given lives? All things being equal and there is no cogent reason why they shouldn't be!

Know it that, in as much as it may sound or be so nice to celebrate things as Christmas, birthdays, new years etc. such acts create unnecessary stress to the brainwaves while all you really sort after is nothing more than: simple momentary joy and harmony. Sure those occasions are great and marvelous to celebrate them but, you should celebrate often in order to savor the positive effect that can be derived from celebrating and feasting everyday and at all times.

Regularity, punctuality with sincerity of purpose is traits that evenly create warm wave of harmony in our brain chips. Such are the benefits we sort after whenever we celebrate; period!

I hereby recommend to all nations to adopt policies that shall make it possible for every citizen to celebrate and feast at a regular and chosen time of the day as we have with the rest of our human activities. That will give too much motivation and enthusiasm for life among every citizen of every sovereign nation of the world. This will also promote unity, love and harmony with an unshakable sense of patriotism!

FOOD AND FEEDING

-GOOD EATING HABIT FOR ALL GLOBAL CITIZENS-

Food, yes! The life-giving substance; any material especially solid taken into the body and assimilated for purposes of growth, nourishment and ideas.

Food as air is next to life; no Food and Air, no life! To entire living creatures including humans,' food provides on daily basis to every one of them, all the energy they will need to activate the smooth functioning of their entire body organs for: moving, eating, talking, and working etc. No one can sustain life for long without food and water, apart from the air that is free and compulsory!

-Notwithstanding, many people have adopted what we refer to as a 'bad eating habit' – eating at random without giving sufficient time for the first food intake to go through complete digestion processes; and also, eating and indulging excessively. This kind of habit also hampers in most cases the real motive for food intake. It is note-worthy for people to know and understand that, it is neither an obligation nor really necessary to eat three square meals daily in order to remain healthy and happy.

-Food as for all other things of creation have got their negative and positive sides; the same food which we work hard every day to have; as nice and as life-saving as they can be, happen to be amongst the top killers in this world of people and animals.

-Most of the known diseases that usually attack humans come from food-intake; imagine the unfriendly odor of a rotten or spoilt food; your feces or excrement; the acidity in your urine; imagine how devastating those can be! Therefore, good health and happy living is not about how much you eat but how well; as I said earlier, everything concerning life and humans, can only yield best results when done with   discipline and in a balanced state of mind. Eventually, with self-discipline, in most cases some of us discover ways to eat correctly by adopting at will, what we refer to as 'a good eating habit'.

A balanced person listens to the ways his/her body reacts to every food intake and unconsciously records the feelings he or she usually obtains after feeding on anything. This is because everything that concerns humankind in relation to his growth, is constantly noted or experienced through the aid of the intangibles known as 'feelings'

-To actually eat healthy in accord with each ones private taste or 'gusto' there is the need to listen to the 'feel'; how you feel after eating whatever it is that you may eat. You should keep taking note of your favorite food intakes; relying on how your body system assimilates or rejects them. By so doing, with time you will arrive at a sound selection of food that your body system likes most and feels comfortable with.

When you are able to achieve that, you should then be able to allow those to be the food you will be eating or feeding on most of the times that you will need to feed.

-Never eat because others do eat or force yourself to eat at the time they do if your body will not be comfortable with the food at that moment; it is not wise to eat such things or at such times that will cause discomfort to your digestive systems or organs.

-Always allow space and time in your stomach before pumping in more food. Eat only when you are really hungry and at regular interval, not to just eat because there is food and it looks appetizing.

-Learn to eat very sparingly; always empty your bowels every morning before starting new food intakes and brush your teeth as many times as you may deem necessary.

-You should in reality brush your teeth and tongue each time you smell rotten food in your mouth and that should be as many times as is necessary- mostly whenever you eat any dairy products, chocolate and sugary things.

-Most people do not care much for their teeth and breath, all they care is eat, drink and smoke without maintaining the organs that make eating possible – teeth, tongue and mouth as a whole should be the part of the body organs that should be treated with utmost respect and care plus the 'bowel cleansing' through a regular and daily excretion.

-Know that to eat healthy does not mean to eat more, worst of all is eating at random. -There is nothing unhealthier to the body than eating at all times- suffocating the metabolic system without allowing it an adequate spacing to successfully finish its initial work of digestion.

-Eat a bit too much or too less for long, your body system will equally react negatively. Your main job as humans is to always find the balance in any venture at all times including in your eating habit.

Punctuality and regularity; those are some of the positive ingredients of entire universal life. Nature does not make much room for over-indulgence; over-indulgence weakens the soul and suffocates willpower.

Every human that eats must as a matter of universal duty and obligation, be able to contribute in food production. Every human is supposed to produce their own food and shelter if all things should be made to remain equal; as in conformity with creational rules devoid of manipulation and adulteration!

SEX AND SEXUAL ORGANS

-SEX AND SEXUAL ORGANS MUST BE TAUGHT OPENLY TO ALL-

Sexual organs are the most fundamental human organs; yet, many do not talk about them freely with joy and appreciation. They are rather treated with scorn; as dirty and things that should always be kept secret.

I think it is stupid for us to be adorned with such important and indispensable organs without using them freely with joy and pride for which they are worth.

The female oval shaped sexual organ biologically known as vagina; and the rocket or bullet-shaped male sexual organ similarly known as penis, are the two most important human organs after the heart and a sound brain. Through them we are able to urinate without which we will run into deadly complications; through the combined actions of the two opposite sexual organs, we are able to consummate sexual intercourse which results into pregnancy and child-bearing; and of course aiding the continuity of species and their races, without which there will be a definite extinction of all created creature in just a few year time space!

We must therefore try to respect our sexual desires with love and affection and do make honest effort to consummate our respective sex-drives in freedom, gratitude and appreciation.

The ex-IGPH students will find a most acceptable way for the public to talk about and treat 'sex-matters'. I suggest we must exclude the irrational talks of morality and religious sentiments attached to people's sexual feelings.

Parents owe a grand duty to teach their respective children the true functions of sex and sexual organs with natural and open mind without the present sense of bias and remorse.

Sex is a word with many definitions: it could simply refer to the two muscular organs located between the two thighs of a person or animal at the lower part of the body which is usually used for urinating and sexual gratification.

Apart from urinating and sexual gratification, every sex organ is also used for child-birth and menstruation particularly for the female genders. 'Sex' as a word could also be used to refer to individual gender: femininity or female; masculinity or male sex organs. *But here, in this book, the word sex will be used to refer to the act of copulation: introducing the male's warm and erect penis into the female's warm, soft and oval shaped vagina with the aim to realize sexual gratification between both of them.* This very act of copulation or sexual gratification is these days than ever being wrongly sought after between men and women of varying age groups.

The gratification or pleasure derived from sexual intercourse between a man and a woman is most of the times so deep and satisfying that many people crazily search for it in such uncontrolled manners, which thereby makes the act itself, very inimical to the senses of equilibrium and mental balance.

Many people as a result also, have resorted to taking advantage of their sexual organs for economic gains through practicing such acts as prostitution, raping, pornography etc.

These days, it had become very trendy to commercialize and abuse sex under various socially accepted names such as:

-homosexuality – the act of having intercourse between man and man or woman and woman instead of the natural way which is between a man and a woman for the main aim of reproduction and multiplication of our human population for the sake of continuity.

- prostitution – which is the act of accepting money or any other form of material gains in order to have sex or make love with the same or opposite sex.

-Pornography – which is the act of allowing oneself to be filmed or videoed making love to oneself (referred to as masturbation) or to another with the final aim of material gains.

-Rape– the act of having sexual relation with another by applying force or violence; which in most cases, ends up in brutal killing, kidnapping, and even mutilation of the body of the raped.

However, let it be known that the main functions of the sex organs are:

-To have pleasure making love between a man and a woman

- To urinate.

-To menstruate and finally:

-To bear children. Any other thing apart or outside these is considered immorality or sexual abuse in the face of most men and the Creator!

The only acceptable sexual conduct in the sight of God and man is an intercourse carried out under the influence of love; provoked by going through the gradual processes of courtship and courtesy in bid to conquer the opposite sex, as to willingly succumb to sexual consummation between the two opposite people. This kind of sexual gratification must be preceded by communication, admiration, respect and with abundant kisses with deepest feelings to be remembered!

As a result, for any marital relationship to be considered successful adequate and satisfactory sexual intercourse must remain a fundamental factor because it is very necessary to lubricate the 'tensions and chains' of daily human affairs.

Well consumed sexual intercourse carried out with deep love affection is a sound mental and physical elixir. It is on the other hand also a panacea to: stress, depression and dissatisfaction – so go for it ladies and gentlemen!

I should encourage the world to take love, sex and sexual intercourse as serious as the food that we eat and air that we breathe.

Forced sexual intercourse does not give real satisfaction to any sane human. In a similar way, when children are born out of deep love, they usually live and behave with much mental balance and maturity throughout their life time; willingly accepting everything about this world with admiration, respect and appreciation. On the contrary, even the parents of such children born without deep and harmonious sex affairs are usually found wanton in the way they behave both as kids and as adults and their conducts are usually unpredictable.

Therefore, sexual intercourse with loving heart and sexual intercourse without loving heart which will you favor most and encourage? Send your answers and comments over this fundamental topic!

EXERCISES

-MIND AND BODY EXERCISE MUST BE MANDATORY TO ALL HUMANS-

What is exercise?

Exercise is the act of voluntary or involuntary engagement of body and soul into activities that heat up the muscles and organs causing the heart to accelerate its beat and also, the blood circulation; this in turn, will help to boost body and soul relaxation as well as boosting the feeling of well-being.

If there is any, there may not be many people out there who do not wish to possess an excellent health and the feel of well-being. It is humanly natural for every individual to secretly wish and desire to appear and be seen as gorgeous, strong and healthy.

But, the big question is- how many people in this modern world are able to reach that goal particularly through their personal initiatives, without external assistances or someone else helping them out?

How many people are able to maintain a sound and stable health for so long on a row without any form of external assistance?

How many people understand and truly believe the fact that: everything about their respective health, state of well-being, freedom of all kind and their happiness, solely lie in their hands?

From experience and from the look of things, many people are not aware of these facts and few are very much aware of it but reluctant enough or unable to combine the stress and grind of regular exercises with the present modern lifestyle: of working in a closed office buildings; and sitting behind a computer for hours on a row, or standing on their feet for hours on a row manipulating machines and other such related jobs. Fact remains that, by the time they leave their respective places of work and get home, they will surely be conquered by fatigue; mostly because of constant routine than of real tiredness.

In a few of such cases, some of the people will be willing to make some exercises to subdue the acquired stress and boredom but will unfortunately discover that their inner spirit is not enthusiastic enough to go along with their bodily need. "The body willing but the spirit very weak" as the saying goes!

At the end, it will be better and nice to sit your butt in your swivel-chair, in front of your Computer (being served and entertained by Microsoft, Goggle and the rest of service providers) for all day working in an office. But the only problem is that type of lifestyle does not help your blood circulation and the enhancement of your body muscles; if you should continue to sit behind a computer for long without warming up your blood, you will never be well enough, such a lifestyle maybe very detrimental to the smooth functioning of your body and mind. To maintain a good health and long life in general, you must always do things that really warm up your blood to aid free circulation or sweat your entire body.

Experience shows that nearly all human possesses that secret desires

to do their very best for themselves; to be the very best that they could afford to be. They all desire to live long and never to die prematurely; and also have the very best of all material possession possible that they could afford to have.

But the big question is- at the end of the day, how many people do truly realize these goals to their very satisfaction? The proliferation of gyms and spa, hospitals and pharmacies plus places of worship of varying categories is a clear demonstration of that strong inner and secret desire of all to get better and to have the best out of life. But, unfortunately, from the look of things- the large number of sick and unhealthy people all around the corner; the large number of people with problem of obesity, anorexics or bulimia; and the large number of people fanatically and devotedly seeking spiritual salvation through prayers at all cost, in a nutshell, clearly shows that "many are truly called but few are truly chosen" as the holy bible said years back!

The above premise makes the wise to understand that many people do not know enough of themselves because, the true meaning of knowing oneself also goes in context with knowing the kind of food that is good for one's stomach to digest better for maximum benefit to one's entire body system.

Entails also, knowing how to gradually nurse your body, your soul, do your daily work, exercise at the same time and keep a positive mind to achieve that secret desire of having the best and being the best that you would like to be and have. These things are the gift of nature for all to possess, there is no magic to it except that of learning to acquire wisdom and keeping a positive mental attitude which harmonizes the forces of nature to make things work out as though with magical sticks.

GOOD NEWS!

The good news is: whenever anyone learns to understand, control and balance his or her mind's composition, his or her eating, playing and working habits will tend to naturally get better; and then, that person's life will begin to assume a dramatic change toward the possible best– enthusiasm for life and for doing positive things will usually begin to rush back to that person from out of some hidden compartments.

Under such positive mental attitude: you will begin to feel that you can do those things that were like impossible to you before; automatically, you will begin to feel that yes, you can do it and do it right. You will start to train your body and soul according to your own natural pace without need to rely on a coach, weights or any other form of external methods or things which are not originating from within you.

This is one of the ways of natural rewards for those who appreciate themselves and things they have already. At that stage, you find out that you will begin to cut down and save on doctor's bills because you have started to run your things well and you have learnt to be your own master coach and your own mentor. These things are simple for those who have faith and confidence in themselves; and to them, gradual and positive changes will start to occur in their respective lives in simple magical succession.

MUSIC AND SOUND

-MUSIC, DANCING AND SINGING SHOULD BE ENCOURAGED-

Music and harmonious sound is a very positive thing for the mind. Music ranks among the greatest gifts of nature duly intended by the Creator to thrill and awaken every kind of human spirit as and when the occasion demands. Above all, it never fails to permeate rich and positive vibration at all times everywhere it is played, heard of or listened to.

A dictionary defines music as-"a combination of sounds which express ideas or emotions by the use of rhythm, melody etcetera".

True, everyone possesses the natural instinct to express ideas and emotions. Everyone is capable to hum, whistle, sing or shake the body in response to emotion. Everyone with or without sight and ears are also capable to read and listen to the ideas or message or emotion delivered through music.

Music is part of human nature and has always been there in different categories from time immemorial.

There are today infinite names of known and unknown musicians from every nook and cranny of the world; so also, there are infinite list of recorded music in the world today which can be listened to or watched through various devices made for music to motivate and elevate the soul and the spirit of mankind to higher dimensions.

But, the thing of interest here is that, upon all that mentioned activities, functions and benefits of music in general, a large number of people still find it hard to dance, sing or express musical feelings without shyness and inhibitions. Only few people usually respond to the beat of music; some do it well enough because they take music as a profession and therefore, practice often; some with mixed feelings of shyness or inhibition, as a result they are unable to express and show their emotions as and how it is being felt deep-down-within them.

Worst still, a good number of people do not express or show open emotions to music whatsoever. They rather expend their positive energy suppressing than expressing the emotions of music which they naturally feel and hear within them.

It is a crime against oneself considering the various numbers and categories of recorded music within everyone's reach to see people not in a position to give at least ten- minutes of one's time out of twenty four hours in a day, to listen, dance or hum to music. Everyone needs some doses of music- dancing, singing and laughing on a daily basis. That also, may require only a bit of discipline to attune ones mind to it.

Dancing and singing to any form of music is recommended as a sound-health tonic. It is a very good therapy both for the mind and for the soul. It makes you feel like a child each time you are riding the sound of music and deep in it! Why not keep 'boogying' with it then, if so good it feels?

THE FEMALE HUMAN SPECIES

-MORE RESPECT AND LEADERSHIP RESPONSIBILITIES-

In conformity with this new era of things-the female human species should be allowed or given the chance to head most political organs of the government in terms of supervision and management. While the male specie will have to mostly assist in all administrative and governmental affairs but, can notwithstanding, be allowed to head and man the rest of the duties that may require more physical energy.

From the look of things and because men had always being there from the beginning; imposing, commanding and managing most things of creation up to this day, and since nothing in life is permanent, we think it will be appropriate also to make a change in the order of things of creation by reversing that unfair notion of male superiority and supremacy over the female genders of this world.

If we knock off pride and superstition and honestly compare men and women in order of services rendered that enriches human life and things; setting examples with instances of pregnancy, family building and positive vibrations surrounding each family atmosphere etc. we will unequivocally conclude the fact that, women are no less superior in no way whatsoever to their male counterparts!

In a normal family set-up; the man wakes from bed every morning, takes his cutlass or other similar farming tools to work. But, these days instead, drive his vehicle to work- to bring food home and with that his job for the day is done in most cases. Meanwhile, the woman is always there from dawn keenly busy with every family member and house chores; she shoulders as well the inconveniences of nine months pregnancy, through to child birth, nursing and feeding each child all through to adulthood; shopping, cooking and caring for all family members all through her life.

She is in most cases, responsible for the house shores and orderliness. Above all, manages to support an arrogant and immature-man; showering everyone with love and well wishes with that constant smile on her 'angelic face'; she seem to be always coated with burning desires for: love, peace, harmony and progress!

They show maturity and discipline which are the basic qualities required for the future global leaders! The female gender in vast majority possesses those cosmic acceptable qualities of positive character trait. Again these days, above all the aforementioned duties vested on her shoulders, she still takes up normal employment as men do apart from administering the whole family affairs which, in my view, carries more work than the 'money-businesses'.

I am hereby solemnly suggesting that we should return the mantle of leadership to the female genders because it is their natural and inherent birth-right. For peace, unity and harmony's sake, we must give this notion a trial; at least. We need to consider the fact that men, mostly, have been for so long in this business of leadership, power and authority; yet our world seem to be negatively progressing instead of positively moving forward.

The ex-IGPH students will have to really look into this important notion so as to come up with the best possible option in support of this laudable vision.

MARRIAGES AND DIVORCES

-NO MORE DIVORCES AFTER MARRIAGE VOWS-

WHAT IS MARRIAGE?

Marriage is an agreement between two opposite sexes with a common aim to live and forever share things and their of lives in general; explore and exploit the pleasures of sexual relationship for the main purpose of reproduction and multiplication which will aid universal continuity for humanity.

If the above premise is accepted to be correct, therefore, all ceremonies attached to marriages are really not necessary ingredients of marriage. And to this very context, it is obvious that most countries in the world have adopted all sorts of superstitious practices with which to express and consummate this unique natural act of love, sex and reproduction which is solely responsible for the continuity and regeneration of entire human race!

The religious organizations have specific rules and conditions that have got to be observed and followed for all their members or adherents in order to be legally accepted as being married! – The Roman Catholic, Muslims, Hindus, Tribal and Civil marriages etcetera have got their norms for legalizing a marital relationship. All those organs reserve their respective views and opinions regarding marital relationships over moral, social and material conducts for all their true adherents.

From the natural point of view; before a couple decides to go into marital relationship, before coming together as one in God and half of each other, they usually must have being courting one another for a while. In most cases, in and out of bed practicing 'pre-sex' before the final decision to be married; all such acts are normal.

But, the only unfortunate situation is the high rate of divorce and separation cases we do encounter daily these days, why? What is supposed to be the causes of these rampant divorces, especially in the technologically advanced countries of the world?

WHAT IS DIVORCE?

Divorce is disavowing or nullification of the oath of marriage; or the breaking of agreement between two people to live and share their lives together forever.

WHAT THEN ARE THE MAIN CAUSES OF THESE RAMPANT DIVORCES?

-From the look of things; it is observed that a good number of marriage agreements were usually contracted with a lot of misgivings due mostly to lack of adequate knowledge or experience at the very moment to embark upon that life changing journey.

- Many people, almost all people are not able to determine the extent of the burden and responsibility that living and sharing one's life with someone else could carry. Because, by meeting someone with whom to 'tango' and establish an intimate relationship and possibly go into marriage, had always being a casual and spontaneous affair. There are no mapped-out rules or ways to go about those kinds of things except by personal instincts and casual intents. No social or moral rules to seek and find a marriage partner outright.

-As a result, many chose what you may term as wrong or improper partners whose relationships tend to end quicker.

-Some people allow meetings to be arranged between them due to cultural, traditional or social reasons; while many others meet through normal process of courtship before taking the decision to be married to one another; fine, all that is fine enough.

But unfortunately, mostly in the recent years, there is no day that passed without something going wrong somewhere in a matrimonial home of one or two people. It is the news of the day carried out as usual by majority of our News Media: divorces, separations, alimony, mal-treatment and sometimes homicide or physical injuries taking places in some marriage homes etcetera. In fact, causes of divorces are innumerable because nearly every culture observes what they consider standard moral and social conducts between couples regarding to marriages; and of course, consequently seek divorces whenever they feel to discontinue or cannot live up to the marriage vows.

In my view, the main causes of divorces in marriages are:

- Ignorance of nature's intention regarding reproduction and multiplication – you do not have to be married to reproduce and aid continuity of humankind in this world; it's your natural gift or assignment as a living being just like the rest of the living creatures, starting from insects to animals.

- Over or under-esteem of oneself; pride, fear and arrogance causes so much havoc in any family where they are harboured.

- Lack of sense of responsibility – being unable to stand by your vow is a kind of betrayal whatsoever your reason maybe; you can't take an oath, a vow to something you can't maintain even in adversity. It's same as irresponsibility. If you can't keep your vow, don't be in marriage. Simple!

- Greed, selfishness and avarice – it is naturally difficult to live and share appropriately together with someone with the above vices. Without the ability to freely give and share, smooth relationships between two people will be hampered and jeopardized.

- Long hours at work by parents – The social obligation imposed on parents through long working hours does not actually help most to concentrate on their children's moral and family education. It is natural that when a man or woman spends many hours at monotonous and boring daily activities, coming home and exhausted; it will be hard to give an adequate and sound attention to the affairs of the family.

- Long hours at school by children – It is alright to go to school, but, because the parents have to also spend lengthy hours at work leaving their children's faith in the hands of strangers as teachers, friends or relatives; at the end of the day, what happens in between going and coming back from school in most cases neither parents nor teachers could be in a position to give a valid account of those hours in between, and all that, does not aid marriage relationship and build a happy family when the child is out of control.

- Selfishness among some couples - no doubt between two people it will take a lot of understanding to live, work and do all their things with the same spirit of oneness and togetherness. The moment any of these two begin to think more of self, things will surely begin to go wrong on the long run and this is also, one of the major reasons of divorces or marital separations.

- Dishonesty and infidelity among others seem to be the most prominent. Once suspicion and uncertainty sets into the mind of one of the couple; the usual enthusiasm and warmth between both couple will tend to dampen and gradually quarrel will set-in; this is human nature. Those with a bad temper will start breaking plates, tearing photos and destroying things which once were of value to both of them.
- What about a violent and jealous husband or wife who derive undue pleasure feasting, hurting and destroying each other with all their respective abilities?

The lists of things that can go wrong in a marital life are too many to account for in a short book of this nature. Irrespective of our human perception of the so called marriage relations, what then is the appropriate way to go about marriages and marriage relationships? Is it naturally necessary to be married in the first place for the world of human race to continue to multiply and go ahead with their lives here on Mother Earth?

NATURE'S INTENTION FOR MARRIAGE

In marriage, the final aim or the natural intention for a man and a woman to agree to live together, is no other than to explore and experience each other's sex organs, share everything and assist each other to build a family full of children and hope. That should be the human intention for going into marital relationships! But to fulfil nature's project for reproduction and multiplication of human race; to aid the smooth continuity of humankind, as it is for the rest of living and non-living things of creation, is marriage vows and relationships a true prerequisite? My answer is no!

But today, nowadays, those main motives do not seem to be the issue any more. People no more think of marriage relationship as a way to bear and raise children; create and build a lasting family. Most marriages do not put that into primary consideration at the moment to tango. Instead, wedding-rings, wedding- dresses, roses and personal interest and material aggrandizement coupled with grand and ostentatious marriage ceremonies largely overshadow each of the couple's minds. As a result, marriage is no more for love-sake and to build a united, disciplined and culturally enriched family which was supposed to continue to maintain human populace of their kinds. That gross act of omission or commission by mankind is making a big mess of this fundamental act of marriage; most marital homes are regularly being broken with their devastating effects over nature's sense of harmony. There are lots of human reasons responsible for these marriage failures.

MAJOR REASONS MOST MARRIAGES FAIL TO STABILIZE

- Most people go into marital relationship, instead of concentrating both of their forces on building love and sound children to aid the prosperity of their family, they rather concentrate their positive energy on building wealth and fame at the expense of Nature's intention for marriages or smooth human relationships!

- Most go into marital relationship, instead of concentrating both forces on learning to understand themselves better, share ideas, plan and work together towards a single goal for both of them, and for the family in general.

- Our justified and accepted social obligations rather tend to put most marriages asunder rather than binding them together.

- Today, every parent spends hours at a monotonous work away from home; their children spending most of their precious time at boring schools in the hands and care of strangers as teachers, maids and friends. But then, we all agreed that "charity should begin at home" in which way could you truly impart and impact on your children so that they will grow up in your image and deeds, if you were never there to educate them with what you know or give to them whatever you have got, talent wise and other-wise?

-The questions are – does doing things in these ways; truly represent those charitable homes worthy of emulation which we fight and aim to achieve?

-Does those ways fulfil and comply with that natural or divinely intentions and purposes of raising rich and happy families? Answers are no.

As in many other aspects of life, the value of marriages and rearing families is being daily wrongly misinterpreted, due mostly to the same ignorance of the creator's intentions for man and woman to tango or due to outright disobedience of cosmic laws of things of creation.

It is because of all these wrong interpretations and values of marital relationships that we have these rampant cases of divorce, alimony, separation, single mothers/fathers; these have become a household vocabulary. Indirectly also, for those reasons - abortion, abandoned children, depression, loneliness, prostitution, infidelity, betrayals are on the increase; for the same reason also, the direct fruits of such unstable families produces: disobedient, angry and undisciplined children who are emanating like locust out of such marital homes.

Are those the charitable homes we vowed and promised to uphold till death during the time to tango and marriage engagements?

How do you think you can make or raise rich, healthy, happy and loving families with those inherited or acquired vices?

My view is that, it will be really impossible if we fail to see marriages as man-made obligations and to place love as a prime factor before making children between you. You have no obligations to make children or be married if you do not do it with heartfelt love!

TRANSPORTATION AND AUTOMOBILES

-Free Global Transportation for all Global Citizens-

Is there any reason why humans cannot permit 'free transportation services for entire fellow global citizens?

Without iota of doubt, the very invention and advent of automobiles is among others, one of the most important technological achievements by human race. We are all aware of and conversant with the numerous kinds of transportation mechanisms in the wide wild world today, ranging from: Bicycles, Motor Cycles, Tricycles- (like the Indian Rickshaw), Quads, Auto-Cars, Buses, Trains, and Airplanes to Ships etc. Any of the above transport medium, will 'jolly-ride you around; some across oceans and clouds' so, permit me to use this medium to thank and congratulate the inventors and manufacturers of all those transport systems, which, have in so many ways improved human's and all forms of life on earth, as well as, their living conditions that have improved extraordinarily due to such laudable inventions!

Didn't humans survived those eras when there was no motor transportation?

Humans survived and very well when there were no motor based transportation and their lives propelled smoothly with a tremendous survival instinct more pronounced than that of the modern people!

Certainly, all humans are made to survive under any kind of condition or situation; no era of humans that have been marked with ease and absolute peace or harmony. In this present time is no exception; we are still living an era of pure stress and struggle for nearly all things irrespective of our automobiles which were made to ease and better our human lives; we are in continuous struggle for survival whether out of man-made or nature-made situations.

In the olden time when there were no auto-transportations, we could walk for days covering distances and getting most things done well even at then. However, we should recognize how tedious and tiring that walking for long distances could be; nevertheless, walking is recommended for the good it does to our dear health.

For the love of unity, peace and harmony of this new order of things in the world, **I hereby suggest and endorse for free transportation systems for all humans; and with the following backup reasons:**

-Vehicles were invented to aid and assist people to move from one point to the other, carry goods and objects of varying dimensions, all in bid to relief the former strain of walking on foot for hours and days to a given destination; also, relief the burden on beasts that were usually transporting heavy loads for us such as: donkeys, horses etc.

-Vehicle uses are making it possible for families to live far away from each other and still communicate regularly whenever and wherever they want.

-Vehicle uses have helped humans a lot in reaching and developing rural areas which otherwise, will be unreachable by any other means. In fact, without the invention and use of vehicles and other machineries, human history today would have being different.

- Obviously, the invention and the use of vehicle has become next to human nature.

Unfortunately, the obvious jolly-ride which vehicles were supposed to give to humans is now being converted into a nightmare instead.

-Vehicle prices are so irrationally exorbitant that billions of world citizens are unable to own, buy, or use any.

-Vehicle ride is so dangerous that millions of humans die regular on daily basis, even as I'm writing and as you are reading, someone is dying somewhere in the world right now from vehicle related accidents.

-Vehicle usage dramatically increased every level of imaginable crimes ranging from: wars, kidnapping, car-bombing, drug trafficking, sexual abuse and human-trafficking; the list of negative and positive activities which the use of vehicles have enhanced, are innumerable.

-Vehicle stress related situations are too much to talk about: beginning from their complicated manufacturing processes to registration, licensing to the constant pollution it carries all along.

-Then come down to the vehicle owner who is obliged to go to driving school, learn synchronized driving styles, road and sign-boards; registration of vehicle on their names, pay exorbitant prices which they are obliged to spend all their life paying without end.

-Vehicle Insurance, "who really invented that 'leech' or blood-sucking vampire"? It is one of the most annoying forms of organized crime with open intimidation! Why not accept certain amount of money on a given vehicle and that will be it; instead of making people pay through all their lives just to own a deadly vehicle? Why do you love money more than yourselves? It is a shame on humans; and disappointing to the Creator of all things which, we have and use today as ever before! Know it that nothing really belongs to any of us; for everything we have is borrowed; and for this premise, I hereby suggest that-**Vehicle use should be free for all human races!**

How could that be done?

-The ex-IGPH students will setup a **'Global Headquarters for all Vehicle-Brands'** that will have to legally approve or permit the manufacture of any vehicle-brand designed by any manufacturer from any part of the world.

-Vehicles being such a fast and vast mortal weapon, despite their best major services to humanity; before any of their manufacture or production: the vehicle's design, security and safety standards of it must be met by the vehicle manufacturers through certified approval from the **'Global Headquarters for all Vehicle-Brands'** (GHVB).

- All vehicles whether small or big must be incorporated with 4wheel-drive for easier and safer access to all terrain.

- We should henceforth stop the manufacture of small cars; fortify the strength and security levels of those approved for production and public use.

-One vehicle only will be permitted for every couple and their children; single people have not much need for a vehicle; they should make use of the free public transport services

-All public transportation networks should be arranged from the global headquarters and distributed to the remotest part of this earth. Even car-rental businesses will be handled by the GHVB. (The modus operandi shall be designed later on)

-Vehicle manufacturers must sell their manufactured vehicles directly to the GHVB under agreement; that then shall embark on the vehicle sale and distribution to the general public according to the set standards.

-Every region or city must have their central representatives who will be attached to the directives of GHVB, making transportation available at all time of the clock to the services and needs of the people of that said region.

To what advantages are these transport regulations in this new order of things?

-To reduce to the barest minimum, the number of people dying daily all over the world, caused by vehicle accidents of varying degrees.

-To reduce the psychological stress caused by such factors as: buying, owning and maintaining a vehicle; most people are forced to buy a vehicle because of work-demands – maybe where you live is not easily accessible to public transport-stands; time of work-fixtures and all such situations. Others want to own a car to show-off and please their ego-demands; etcetera.

-However, the above reasons to own a car cannot compensate for the: pollutions from the vehicles which you use, the city congestion, the accidents, the noise… we will make sure that people go wherever they want and whenever through providing adequate services to encourage people to sacrifice for the new system of things for the sole benefit of all of us!

BUSINESS AND NORM

-MORE TIME TO FAMILY AND NATURE; LESS TIME TO BUSINESS AND MONEY-

What is Business?

Business is simply: the act of doing anything whatsoever for economic rewards.

Looking down from the past human history and to these present global political dispensations, it's obvious that majority of human race spend almost all their precious time in pursuit of economic rewards and material gains.

Why do Humans Chose to Spend Most of Their Precious Time for Material Aggrandizement against Self and Universal Knowledge?

Is that the best way you can discover to make you feel good and at peace?

How could you deliberately give away for so little as 'money', most of your precious and invaluable time which is naturally given to you to do all your things for yourself and for those around you; things for yourself as: reasoning in silence by yourself and your Creator, meditate in open and with clear mind, give time to also study about yourself and try to know the real you and what you do really want out of this conglomerate and infinite abundance of 'Mother Nature'.

With a bit of wisdom and deeper knowledge of sound living, you will perceive the futility of taking yourselves too serious while in normal pursuit of your dreams and aspirations in this very life that we are living. You should rather strive to pursue your goals and aspirations with high enthusiasm, humility and joy from the challenges they usually offer or carry along with them. Know it that, whatever you may invent or create today or tomorrow to come in this very world, will only serve to bring 'just joy of that moment in time'. Everything, together with their respective rules for individual and co-existence had long been stipulated, created and concluded!

Your main purpose in life is nothing more than making good use of all that which nature abound for your entertainment; while you grow and ultimately die and rot away'.

When you learn enough to perceive your own life, those of others, you will then surely, know that the only realistic joy derivable out of all elements of life is: the act of sharing and giving; sharing unconditionally with enthusiasm everything you have got, from ideas, jokes to material things.

Such attitude to life adds enormous benefits to your body, mind and soul.

Know it also, that, obsessive accumulation of material things by a nation or person, is a plain sign of ignorance and of course, of fear of lack and pride; more things you have, more problems of stress you will equally accumulate in proportion and which, will ultimately compound your very simple existence. Do away with most things that are inimical to unity, peace and happiness of your soul.

Therefore, make more effort to select businesses that give you joy instead of stress and sleeplessness.

This being so, it is therefore stupid to spend your precious time in vain pursuit of money and material aggrandizement.

Henceforth, we should enact and design fair laws that will enable humans to spend more time and make most effort to build rich, healthy and happy families. We should take our lives more serious as more precious than gold and silver for which it really is. Question is: *will it be better for you to have all the wealth in this world at the expense of your unique health and life?* My own answer is absolutely, NO! Send your own answers and comment to these views, please.

Without a sound health, your money and businesses are useless to you of course; so, why all these craze, betrayals, and anxiety for money and businesses; what sense is there in all that much ado at family and self expense?

Think my people; reason! As the global community gets wiser, this world will get better and every creational thing and humans will begin to change to their best ever; you will then discover to your dismay that all your accumulated wealth had been a wasted labor; because, with a positive mental attitude to life, wealth and material aggrandizement take the lowest place of significance in the scale of 'life's values' and this is easy to happen in this new era of things; thanks to this new global easy access to information for all global citizens; for that, collectively we owe unreserved gratitude to those behind: Microsoft, Face Book, Google, Yahoo, Twitter and all the rest of the Media-Outlets making it easy to access and share information across the global community at the push or click of a button!

HOUSING AND LAND MANAGEMENT

-Lands and Houses should be Free for all Global Citizens-

No more buying or selling of neither lands nor houses. Lands do not belong to no one at all; lands are the exclusive property of the Creator; just like: seas, stars, moon, sun, sky, the cloud and the air we breathe etc.

Land is just one of those elements of nature created for our collective succor and nurture; land is not a thing to own, it is not a belonging! Unbelievable that we, the global citizens had continued from time immemorial to accept that wrongdoing of buying and selling lands which is exclusive property of the Creator!

It is really ugly and repulsive for humans to engage in such negative actions; no doubt, if you could find a way to do it, you will be buying and selling this air that we breathe, the sea that flows, the stars and moon that shines and the sun that warms and lights all things!

Why is this over anxiety for money and material possession taking hold of entire global community? I feel shame most times for being part of human specie due to their negative attitude and gross sign of ingratitude to the Creator and his creations; forgive me for my outburst!

Here is the best way to use our given lands for unity and equality in this new era of things:

- once a boy and a girl come of age and decide to marry with each other, for such union as a couple, they will be given a pre-mapped piece of land in any chosen community where the said couple will want to live. This will enable them to cultivate the given land, grow their own food, their own house; make children and multiply with peace and harmony.

-Naturally, shelter is the number two most important three basic needs of human beings after food, it therefore beats my every imagination why humans are not able to freely utilize the vast lands naturally given to them for their collective use and for sustenance on earth while they grow, multiply and then, die and rot away; why must they hassle and create unwanted obstacles for each other? Why must they possess what they do not really need while others amongst them have nothing?

-If all the other creatures: animals, insects, fishes, micro and macro-organisms live freely in and on the lands, seas, jungles, air etc, why then must human race be made to pay to own a piece of land to shelter them in order to sustain their existence on Mother-Earth? Does that make any sense to you? Think it over properly; something is definitely wrong with humans for accepting and cherishing such kinds of chaotic ventures.

- Every human family has a birth-right to a piece of land and also, the natural obligation to produce at least one regular eatable item as contribution to Mother-Nature.

- Every human must be given the chance and appropriate coaching on how to produce most of the things that they consume on daily basis such as: rearing animals, planting fruit trees, vegetables or cultivate tubers etc. for it will be a shame and utterly against Mother-Nature for any human to go through life without producing at least one eatable item; such negative trend is inimical to the progress and prosperity of this world. Such conducts is a veritable act of parasitism; blood-sucking leeches and bad weeds in someone's vegetable farm! We can no more tolerate or continue to live our pretty lives as paupers in the sphere of abundance.

- Having all the money and properties in this world without you producing any of the food you eat daily is a wrong presentation; you are not showing a good example to the growing youth. Can you directly eat your money or property? Answer is no! You need food to live in a house. Therefore, you should have known to produce some of the food you and your family will eat everyday to help in nature-building. 'I very well understand the past and present global economic trends; the need in favor of the popular term "Division of Labor" and its connotations; so far so good.

However, the big question remains 'Is this current way we run our society the best approach on how to live with and in Nature for progress and prosperity sake?

To this fundamental issue, the ex-IGPH students will find a way to harmonize such issues as land and housing.

Land and houses must be free for every global citizen and every global citizen on their own or in return must always be in a position to produce at least one edible item wherever they may live; whether in the desert, snow, forest, city and villages! In this new era there will be no excuse whatsoever for any human not to have a place to live nor something to cultivate with money or no money. If we want, yes we can! This time around we all really should want it for peace and harmony to reign supreme everywhere!

SPORTS, ARTS AND CULTURE

-All Humans must Practice any Arts or Sports on Daily Basis –

Why sports, arts and culture? Does it matter to anyone what you do with yourself?

-Truth is, human beings like most other creatures, are structured to go through regular body, mind and soul maintenance with the works that they do or other exercises; in order to remain fit, well and healthy.

-Yes it matters so much to me what you choose or will choose to do with your good self; why? Because, to realistically live a successful and "good life" you must have enough energy reserve. Yes, you need a lot of energy even to be happy, dance well, and laugh well; to play, you need positive energy to do all things. That into perspective, you will agree with me that it is absolute nonsense for anyone to live without sports, arts and cultural practices.

-Know it that, the real food for your mind apart from oxygen and glucose are the intangibles such as: imagination, all physical and mental activities; as well as regular adventures which provides

experiences that in turn aliments and strengthen the neurons that distributes information to all other parts of the body organs. While the physical food that we consume help to aliment our entire body cells which in turn sustain the energy necessary to ignite and run the engine of our life.

In this new order of things, we want to see majority of humans more healthy, happy and prosperous. When you are healthy, you can be happier, impact more positively on others and enjoy more of life with much enthusiasm than when you are weak and ailing.

Do not wait for the doctors, start today to practice any activity of your choice that you can do regularly; prevention is always better than cure; don't you agree any more to that old long sayings. Do not wait to be sick before you can take yourself serious health-wise.

By the way; is there any other thing in your life that is more important than you yourself? Answer is no! If you feel or know yourself to be that important why then neglect your good self always as you presently do?

Activities or any form of physical and mental exercise help in no small measures to fortify your brain-chip, your physical body and all the body organs that sustain the smooth functioning of your entire being; so go for it now for your good and that of our global peace and harmony! When you are healthy and happy, every other thing and people around you will as well in equal proportion be healthy and happy! This is the way we want all global citizens to be and to feel in this new era of our life time! Enough of ill health and poor sense of humor; happiness and good health are free of charge; all you require to obtain them is only but, participation, desire and action!

CHILDREN AND THE FUTURE

-Today's Children will definitely become Tomorrow's Parents and Leaders-

-If you agree with me that these children we see now and today, will definitely become parents and future leaders; the parents and leaders of tomorrow. Why then do we tend to disrespect them and treat their matters without much consideration or as second place citizens?

For example: from years now, we have coined and retained in our global lexicon such phrases as: "You are acting like a child" "you are just a child" what are the literal meanings of such expressions?

Literally, such expressions or phrases could mean that the 'child' or children is/are stupid, nonchalant, or utterly unreliable and not dependable; could also mean that the 'child' is irresponsible and know not how to act appropriately.

All over the world in a similar manner, there are laws based on the ages of children; for example: from which age that children must start and finish schooling; from which age they should be allowed to participate in certain sportive activities; and at what age to drive or smoke or drink…the list of things children cannot do or participate in with their parents or on social levels are innumerable.

- Until eighteen years of age in most European countries, you are considered a child without right to do most things you see your parents do daily such as: drinking alcoholic contents, smoking cigarettes, marijuana or any intoxicant, and even driving or travelling on their own without permissions are not allowed until they are eighteen years of age! In some countries they peg the age at sixteen years before a growing child is considered adult and with rights to do things they desire. And in some other places, children have no written age limits as in Africa or parts of Asia, in such places, to be considered an adult with rights of decision and participation in what assumed adults are doing; the parents or cultural backings determine when their growing children should be duly accepted as grown-up adults! Whatever the reasons, the criteria or motives for backing such laws and attitude toward our beloved children, I have no idea; all I do know is that you are trying to do your best for our beloved children bla-bla-bla.

-I only want to use this medium to bring it to your knowledge that, your approach to the sincere education of our children– global future leaders- is not right, it is not appropriate to discriminate against our children, oblige them always to do things against their will or volition; for example: schooling, driving, use of many things they are not allowed while their parents do and use those things. That is share hypocrisy!

-You should know that, when a given child is imbued with appropriate and sound education, that very child can do so many of those things we ask them not to do even more responsibly than most of the so called adults and parents.

- know it that I have seen, known and lived with children who are more clever than their parents, do their things and comport their lives much better than their parents.

- If we educate our children with the correct stuff in their mind, they will surely behave correctly as soon as they begin to think and reason with adults; which means they can as well do whatever adults are doing if we allow them.

-I feel it is right that we should let our children to begin earlier to experience and discover life by themselves through errors and trials; To protect them from danger is to deny them of the ability to develop their own natural survival instinct and discourage them from life of adventure which is the correct thing to do or the 'proper way to coach a growing child' towards the adulthood.

- I have written a book based on these issues: ('How to Educate Children with Ease').

- I noticed that children begin to use their minds almost fully as their parents from the ages of five upwards. At this age they could as well do whatever the adults are doing; the only difference between a children and their parents is -experience. Experience they must definitely have with activities and getting things done well or wrong… In fact, our children generally prefer to do whatever their parents are doing, they like to and feel they could if allowed. So let's give them that benefit of doubts to make mistakes and learn from their respective mistakes; to be in danger and learn to fight their respective ways out of said dangers.

Why must our children have to be eighteen or be given any age-peg or limit for them to begin doing things that they can rightly do well today and now if allowed? If they have all the bureaucratic red tapes removed for them to listen and follow their heart desires without interferences such that are listed above, they will definitely do and be doing greater things even at such an early age!

BEST OPTION FOR OUR CHILDREN

-MORE RESPECT AND ATTENTION TO GLOBAL CHILDREN-

Do you know that every child is born with their own brain-chip in which, the child's unique characteristics relating to his or her personality trait is deeply engraved?

I believe that a child's personality trait is uniquely transferred through the phenomenon 'DNA' and I also suspect that 'DNA' molecular contents continue to shuffle and reshuffle its data; influenced by time factors, geographical position of the parent at the moment of a child's formation; and probably, influenced by the earth position at the precise moment of a child's formation or conception as it revolves around the sun. Those natural influences or phenomena may usually determine the personality trait of a given person; and also, may rightly answer the question: why our finger prints varies; why every single human have got a unique finger print and as well, why genealogy can be traced through the DNA-match!

Based on the above observations, the ex-IGPH students will have to review the laws governing our children as to modify certain conditions or influences, be it, social or family which, will psychological and physically favor them, their parents and our collective global communities without exception.

If our today's children will become our tomorrow's parents and leaders, it is therefore prudent to invest most of our positive energy and wisdom to make them be and have the best of everything possible that we could offer; with love and affection, and, without any form of reservation. To consolidate that notion I want to invoke the golden rules of nature:-

From the subtle ways of the nature of things of creation; basing on the immutable laws "of give and take", "seek and find", and "to others as you would like them do unto you" for example, I am kind of constrained to suggest that we revise and modify the present global order of work-schedule in such a way as to give enough time to every family to be able to attend to themselves; especially, attend to the children in their respective family. Those children happen to be, by all essence, the foundation stone of the future of this world; they are the tomorrow's leaders and giving adequate time to them is to me a very important long term investment that shall prove to be very beneficial to all and sundry.

The serious business of rearing children to make up a family should be promoted, publicized and given as much attention as is necessary. This will surely enhance deep affection for owning and running a family; and as well, guarantee matured and disciplined children, who should do much better and progressive than we have them today.

Today's children will automatically become tomorrow's parents and eventual leaders! This in mind therefore, it will be quite unwise and imprudent not to give as much time as possible to our given children so as to make the best possible off them.

To achieve that, I will suggest that we give half of our total daily hours to our children; that time input on them, will be gradually fortifying that fundamental sector as a solid part of our global 'future investments'. Because, the more time you spend with your children, the more you are bound to know what kind of stuff or traits they are composed of; their natural abilities and inclination and most importantly, also, you will be able to directly impact and impart to them whatever you have to offer as a parent, outside their teachers and external mentors.

Doing that will give the entire world a better chance to rear children with balanced mental attitude; which is most necessary for any kind of human success and progress.

As best option for our children's sake, I am suggesting also, that we try to adopt a policy where each family should not give more than ten working hours on daily bases to public work or services (between wife and husband). It have to be that, either the woman of each family will have to do five hours of work or services and so for the man as well; or that the man of each family should serve an hour more than the woman if need be; this suggestion is based on the fact that the children usually require the attention of both parents for them to be in a balanced mental attitude; even both husband and wife will require the steady attention of each other to be in a state of balanced and positive mental attitude to make their child rearing duty to blossom.

This kind of project can be enhanced through a system designed to organize – **"Best Family Contest Awards"** on a global perspective. That must somehow encourage families to be doing and giving their very best while bringing up their hard earned children.

We can also, organize other national and regional awards for **"The Best Behaved Child/Children"** as well as **"The Best Parents of the Year Awards"** etcetera. This will encourage parents to be giving their best to their children and vice versa.

It is our collective global duty to make our people understand and to be conscious of the fact that this child-rearing business is the most important aspect of our future lives and should be duly accepted and honored accordingly.

The children and family rearing jobs are globally more important and beneficial to the world at large than those of movie and money makers.

We should try to divide the working hours and schedules into four shifts of five hours work with one hour of break for each shift. This also will have the advantage of allowing more families to have jobs to do as well; instead of one person doing nearly ten hours and above straight at a given job, while others have nothing to do; also the habit

of working for eight or ten hours straight at a given job is detrimental to family relationship, friendship and even to personal health.

If we can collectively on a global perspective design our system of leadership based on these principles from the start of this unique book, that will surely bring back and promote most of the lost values that go with family relationship in general and will also help to minimize the rampant misconduct of children and the disruption of families that took a lot of pain and hard work to find and to build.

This will surely be a huge global input and more profitable for all of us on the long run; will also, enhance the sense of leadership of unity and equality for all humanity!

Thank you for your time and collaboration!

GLOBAL SYSTEM RESHUFFLE

Now is the time for a global system reshuffle! Now is the time for all global people to fully partake in the: social, economic and political administration of every affairs concerning their free given lives.

This present system of human leadership had ceased to be feasible; it had remained out of vogue; it had become archaic. In the past, this same system of leadership had fought brutal wars and conquered territories; made formidable history in varying dimension!

From the past down to this present time, our human system of leadership had continuously being exploring and exploiting everything freely given by nature: the Land, the Sea, the space and environment; also, the human mind and body. In consequence, we have duly created: Icons, Saints, Gurus, and Heroes and Legends nearly in all dimensions or facets!

GENERAL QUESTIONS– *the general question at this moment are: In all the human bravery from the past down to this present time, have we ever found peace and harmony? Are we duly in love and in unity with ourselves and the world around us? Do we have a globalized code which is duly structured to achieve global peace, unity and harmony?*

This book had ventured to structure a globalized system of leadership streamlined in harmony within the dictate of **'Nature and positive natural feelings'**! In essence, there is nothing wrong with this world we live in. But, there is a lot of things wrong in the ways we manage the affairs of this awesome world; living a life is absolutely simple and easy; but, we complicate and mix-up most of the issues of nature due to ignorance. Because of ignorance, we tend to move against the tide instead of flowing and surfing with the tide. For those wrong doings 'Mother Nature' is angry and this present global crisis and austerity is a slight nemesis from nature, for our ceaseless wrongdoing!

Humans, being conceived and born in ignorance, every mistake they make is acceptable; but, it is absolutely unacceptable not to amend and rectify the mistake and move ahead in peace and harmony with our so-short lives here on earth. Now is time for a piece of peace; goddamit!

"Humanity in Disarrays & Ways Forward" is a book duly inspired to achieve global peace, harmony, love and unity amongst all sovereign nations; people and the entire environment! *Now is time for a positive system reshuffle for the good of all!*

NO MORE WARS AND FIGHTING

No more wars; no more fighting; avoid these senseless killings of one another; and also prevent against these undue global contaminations. We are now in the new era of global peace and harmony; now is time to begin to apply the positive 'Golden-Rules' of creation in all our daily global affairs; enough of short-cuts to our given lives; enough of sharp-practices against the stable rules of creation. Short-cuts don't pay well in this distant race for survival; all things gained out of sharp-practices usually flickers and twinkles with instability and eventually crumble!

Know it that any person, group of persons or nation that in others stir strife and confusion will always go down in this very long race for life in time to reckon; and in the similar way, any person, group of persons or nations that give or are giving the most in good services to others will always be rewarded in abundance and remain stronger in this long race for life! Those are some of the infallible 'Nature's Rules'

This book is the founding guideline for the new world constitution for the only possibility of global unity, peace and harmony ever lived in the entire history of human-race! Accept it and treat it with utmost reverence for the good of entire global community.

"Humanity in Disarrays & Ways Forward" is a unique book written under the guidance and influence of divine inspiration. The author has managed to put this book together in a pure state of a 'child's mind' with little or no bias whatsoever. Judging from the book contents many will think or imagine that the author is well read; or had carried out enormous research about the system of things in this world and its citizens that gave him the correct insight and authority to write or delve into these kinds of controversial topics which many people will duly consider as sacred or out of an ordinary human's reach and pondering.

This book was written in absolute solitude and in the midst of multitude without prior knowledge of the actual political, economical, social, academic or technological realities of the world the author lives in; and with the only mission and vision to bring and foster: unity, peace and harmony in the entire world irrespective of race, creed, geographical location and gender.

How could the author have known the real situation of the system of things of the world if he never participated or researched over the actual global system of things? Is it possible he had actually been taught and guided by the Divine Spirit to write a book that is so precise and irrefutable with viable contents that can surely bring unity, love and harmony to global community?

In the author's words: "the illusion to enact laws with which to lead or rule people and the entire world is one of the most lousy and stupid superstition devastating some human's minds". People should give up the unnatural pursuit of leadership of people and things; and if they can do that, this world will run so smoothly for all, so well that you will never imagine possible. Why do you want to make laws above the natural laws intertwined within the creation of all things? Why do you want to rule and control a world which you did not create?

All you are supposed to do as humans is no more than for you to live and let others be and live as well without unnecessary additions and subtractions; period!

Like any modern human, the author has been indoctrinated through the social education system; has been indoctrinated through the religious institution and all the rest of the established institutions of "brain-drain" yet his mind remain unaffected. He has seen his country and his ancestors annihilated and their ideals devastated and thrown into turmoil by those trying to divide and rule others by all means possible, yet, his mindset has remained untouched… in essence, what does that teach us? Think my people, think!

That is a simple indication that, normal people cannot rule and control this world and the mind of people in it without repercussions and great difficulties. In all intent and purposes, few people among humans have being ceaseless trying to dominate and control others from thousands of years without absolute success. They have only succeeded in dividing and ruling with: lies, cheating, hypocrisy, intimidation, suppression, wars, destruction and all forms of mischief.

For the divine sake of unity, peace and harmony of this awesome world of people, plants and animals, can you all now give up that unattainable illusion of supremacy and try to be humane? Doing so will open our minds to show love and respect for every single human, plants and animals instead of: trying to control, subjugate, and deceive; humiliate, kill and slander! Save yourselves all that trouble because you are all created in the same process as everyone else; you are not the Creator therefore, can never ever be in a divine position to manage the mechanism of life and living! Enough of trying to dethrone the Creator and unlawfully take his place; it is an illusion which must be discouraged by all means and in all its essence; you can only achieve disruption colossal collapse of people and things!

NATURE'S LAWS ARE INFALLIBLE

- I AM A LIVING WITNESS-

As a living witness to the **'Infallibility of Nature's Laws**, for having spent all my reasoning life in spiritual battle within my innermost self, toiling day and night to live every second of my daily life in love, faith and harmony with the world around and the two great opposing spiritual forces living inside of me; and metaphorically speaking, 'I have become fully possessed by what we refer to as the Holy-Spirit'.

This book is a testimony of the infallibility of the cosmic laws of creation on the positive side; of which, that humble state of mind can only be attained through thinking rightly, doing things rightly and living rightly in accord with nature's laws; as ingrained in our respective 'minds' from birth up into the wonders of the Creator; and to maturity and decline...

It had always been my childhood-deepest-desire to see this world, people and every other thing inside it, to live as one that it really is; and to live in a world where love, peace, unity and harmony is constantly emanating and oozing out of every human family and relationships. Inspired by such noble desires, every suggestion contained in this book is deeply rooted on years of battle trying to remain in harmony with natures' laws as ingrained and felt from deep-down-within, which had made it possible for me to come to know that, doing things right; for example, by following the suggestions contained in this book will help a lot to bring peace, love and harmony for entire living and non-living matters in this wide-wild-world (www) smile!

Having toiled in the dark and been guided and governed by ignorance – I did not have enough experience as at then, to know what I do know now with the passage of time- I am fortunate or privileged to have learned so much about life or creational lessons out of all that toiling in the dark, resisting most 'man-made-laws' and often landing in the depth of human 'shit' and troubles after the other.

In my ardent search for the precise and best way to live a life that is pleasing and harmonious to: me, my family who I owe much respect; all other creatures as plants, cloud, rain, and insects and above all, to the unseen and silent Creator in whom I'm well pleased; and who, I hold in absolute awe, for the very mystery of 'How it did all began'? (Please close this book at this stage and for ten minutes, try to imagine or visualize – how God or the Creator came into the scene of existence; how was the Creator created? What was the entire space like before creation started; if they say that, there were no light, darkness, atmosphere… before the Creator eventually appeared on the scene of things, so, how did it all began? **Think, please keep thinking!**

In my sincere effort to honor and realize that simple desire to always think, do and live right; I have along the way been: mal-treated, cheated, humiliated, intimidated and often angered to near madness. Even family and supposed friends have abandoned and betrayed me. But, above all that, I refused to quit or renounce my desires; and as a reward for my applied-faith in my belief, **I had been duly awarded a 'spare-key' with which to open at will, the golden gate of love, peace and harmony of which the whole wide-wild-world are scampering for everyday of their lives; and unfortunately, searching on the wrong part to achieve a fruitful existence!**

I hereby use this medium to invite the entire human-race to come together with me, that we can hand-in-hand walk through that 'Golden-Gate' of love, peace and harmony and also, to remain there for a while in brotherhood and sisterhood in all our neighborhoods; With neither more fighting nor rancor and bitterness!

My happiness is this knowledge that "everything pertaining to life as an entity and creation in its entirety, is ingrained deep-down-within our mind's-chip. That makes it easier to manage and control our mind's chip in order to serve us in the best ways possible. This book will and must show you how to think right and act right by following the positive side of your innermost mind; and empowered by the forces of positive desires and deeds.

As a true witness to the infallibility 'of Nature's Laws' I had somehow, traced millions of years of past creational history down to this very present time; and what about the daunting future?

In all those past millions of years of human history, humans have done wonderful and awesome things; and still discovering and trying many other things yet unknown to humanity. But, the most daunting is knowing that in all the long spanning years of human history, we do not yet know precisely, what life is all about; why the phenomenon 'Life' has to exist in the very first place; and what makes life or living so wonderful…bla-bla-bla…

Why so easy? Because everything is in the mind's chip within our respective reach and control; so, what more could humans ask for? We have got ingrained deep down within us all that it take to live in this world, not just as brothers and sisters, or as families in all our communities, but more also, in heavenly peace, love and durable harmony! "YES WE CAN" therefore, LET'S JUST DO IT! WE HAVE GOT ALL IT TAKE TO GET THINGS DONE AND MOVING!

Nature's laws are infallible; you can investigate them yourselves. There is nothing wrong with creation or anything about this world; the Creator had done with creation the most perfect and awesomely mysterious work of all time and space. All human problems are resultant effects of their wrong plans of thoughts and actions taken by them to supplement their given things of life. In a similar pattern, we

can still undo and better the past wrongs man had done to man himself, things, and the Creator. In order to realize that life-changing dream we must reshuffle this entire world through proactive and feasible legislation consciously channeled towards embracing eternal peace, love and harmony for all created creatures within the deep, above and surface of this awesome Earth!

Every single sentence or phrase inside this book is inspired for good; they present the best possible ways forward to guide, appease and relief humanity in total disarrays and near devastation to the point of no return; to the stage of impossible rehabilitation…

WITH HEART-FELT LOVE!

www.ingramcontent.com/pod-product-compliance
Lightning Source LLC
Chambersburg PA
CBHW021014160726
47994CB00006B/2516